Coping Successfully with Shyness

Margaret Oakes is completing her final year of training as a Counselling Psychologist at City University, London and will shortly be registered with the British Psychological Society and UK Health Professions Council. She has experience of providing psychological interventions in primary care and NHS specialist services. Margaret is a consultant with Dynamic Change Consultants, <www.dccclinical.com>, a psychology consultancy in London. Her focus in psychological consultations is to provide tailored evidence based interventions most likely to be effective for the individual clients she works with. She has a particular interest in anxiety disorders. Margaret is also a pilot, currently operating the Airbus A320 series of aircraft for a UK airline.

Professor Robert Bor is a Director of Dynamic Change Consultants, and Lead Clinical Psychologist in Medical Specialties at the Royal Free Hospital, London. He is a Chartered Clinical, Counselling and Health Psychologist registered with the UK Health Professions Council. He is also a Fellow of the British Psychological Society and Member of the American Psychological Association. He has more than 27 years' experience consulting in clinical and organizational settings in the UK and abroad. He is a UKCP Registered Family and Couples Therapist, having specialized in Systemic Therapy at the Tavistock Clinic, London. Rob also practises cognitive behavioural therapy and is an advocate of time limited and solution focused therapeutic approaches. He works with children, adolescents, adults, couples, families and teams in organizations, and is the Consulting Psychologist to the Leaders in Oncology Care and to the London Clinic, both in Harley Street. He also provides psychological consultations and Executive Coaching to organizations such as PWC and UBS among others in London and abroad. He is the consulting psychologist to St Paul's School, The Royal Ballet School and JFS in London. He holds the Freedom of the City of London and is a Churchill Fellow.

Dr Carina Eriksen is a Chartered and UK Health Professions Council Registered Counselling Psychologist with an extensive London based private practice for young people, adults, couples and families. She is a consultant with Dynamic Change Consultants and an accredited member of the British Association for Behavioural and Cognitive Psychotherapies, having specialized at the Institute of Psychiatry. She has managed a team of psychologists, CBT therapists and psychotherapists in the NHS for several years and she used to be an external supervisor at the Priory. She has extensive experience consulting in clinical and organizational settings in the UK and Europe. Carina is a consultant at Colet Court, St Paul's School for boys and she works closely with several British and International schools in London. She is actively involved in research with a specific interest in the topic of work stress and work/life balance anxiety, panic, fear of flying, and the psychological effects of living with cancer. Carina and her colleagues are often invited to present these topics at conferences in the UK and abroad.

Overcoming Common Problems Series

Selected titles

A full list of titles is available from Sheldon Press,
36 Causton Street, London SW1P 4ST and on our website at
www.sheldonpress.co.uk

Overcoming Common Problems Series

Overcoming Common Problems Series

Overcoming Common Problems

Coping Successfully with Shyness

MARGARET OAKES, PROFESSOR ROBERT BOR
DR CARINA ERIKSEN

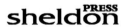

First published in Great Britain in 2012

Sheldon Press
36 Causton Street
London SW1P 4ST
www.sheldonpress.co.uk

The author and publisher have made every effort to ensure that the
external website and email addresses included in this book are correct and
up to date at the time of going to press. The author and publisher are not
responsible for the content, quality or continuing accessibility of the sites.

British Library Cataloguing-in-Publication Data
A catalogue record for this book is available from the British Library

ISBN 978-1-84709-211-3
eBook ISBN 978-1-84709-212-0

Typeset by Fakenham Prepress Solutions, Fakenham, Norfolk NR21 8NN
Printed in Great Britain by Ashford Colour Press
Subsequently digitally printed in Great Britain

Produced on paper from sustainable forests

Contents

This book is dedicated to the many people who have shared with us their experiences of feeling anxious, awkward or shy in social situations. Working with them has given us an insight to the varied and individual ways in which these difficulties have an impact on thoughts, behaviour and emotions. This depth of understanding is the foundation of this self-help book, which we hope will help others to overcome their shyness and anxiety.

1

Why another book about shyness?

Numerous books have been published on coping with social anxiety and shyness, so why have we written another one?

There are several reasons – and this chapter will outline how this book and our approach are different from others. It will highlight tried and tested methods for overcoming social anxiety and shyness as well as unique and specific ones which we hope you will find useful and effective. Our experience with people who have difficulties with shyness or social anxiety shows that, although some books provide useful information about coping with specific situations, such as public speaking, they may not explain the full range of modern psychological techniques which are known to help overcome – or at least cope with – feeling shy, awkward or anxious in social encounters.

Helping you to master these techniques is the main focus of this book: its purpose is to show you how to select and practise the techniques most likely to help you overcome your social anxiety or shyness. We also outline the way in which shyness becomes an issue in the first place, and how different people are affected by it.

Shyness and social anxiety have a significant impact on the personal, family and professional lives of a substantial proportion of the adult population. Published research suggests that around 7.5 per cent or more of the adult population may show clinical symptoms. This is something that many young people and adolescents also experience. It is fair to say that almost everyone has been shy or affected by social anxiety at one time or another, but for some there is a constant battle with anxiety in situations where they encounter other people, whether socially, at work or otherwise. While for some it may be a small annoyance and something which is slightly inhibiting or uncomfortable, for others it may be extreme and result in incapacitating fear that can lead to avoidance of all social situations. This, in turn, may place strain on personal and professional lives. Difficulties in social situations, therefore, should not be lightly dismissed.

Shyness can occur in specific and well-defined situations. It can also affect a person's confidence in a much broader range of contexts, and anxiety, awkwardness, embarrassment and general unease can be some of the symptoms experienced across a range of situations. In extreme circumstances, it may lead to avoidance of all social contact. It can also affect your capacity to form and maintain relationships. It can affect your ability to give – and receive – emotional and social support to or from friends and family, damage careers, spoil holidays and put relationships under stress. The good news is that there are effective skills and techniques which you can use to reduce the fear and anxiety commonly associated with social situations, all of which are described in this book.

Social anxiety and shyness are among the most treatable psychological difficulties. For this reason, almost everyone should be able to overcome this fear – provided that it has been properly assessed and treated using modern psychological methods. This book brings together the latest proven methods for overcoming social anxiety.

What makes this book different?

This book takes an approach to the challenge of overcoming shyness or social anxiety which you are unlikely to see taken in many other books on this topic. There are four main ways in which it is different:

1 It is written by a highly experienced and uniquely qualified team of psychologists who have extensive experience in treating social anxiety and helping people to overcome shyness. We are committed to helping people overcome their anxieties and apply tried and tested methods to achieve this. Each of us is qualified and experienced as a general psychologist, and therefore we have experience in assessing and treating a wide range of psychological difficulties. We also have considerable experience of helping people with the specific issue of social anxiety. We find that almost all psychological difficulties can affect, interfere with or disrupt personal relationships and that living with almost

any psychological condition – such as depression or obsessive–compulsive disorder – can affect your confidence and make you feel self-conscious. We are aware of and sensitive to the impact of social anxiety in people's lives, as well as the sense of shame, embarrassment and fear that so many people experience by having this or other psychological issues. Together, we have more than 40 years' experience. We have published our research findings in specialist medical and psychological journals, as well as in books, and we are often invited to talk about our work at conferences around the world.

2 We approach treatment differently from some others who deal with shyness and social anxiety, and this book reflects that perspective: it will not baffle you with statistics about social anxiety; we will certainly not convey, or focus on, the idea of social anxiety being an irrational fear; we will not 'argue with' or dismiss any fear you may have that may seem illogical or irrational to others (and sometimes even to you!). This book facilitates a tailored approach to self-help, built on a solid foundation of clinical practice and research. The aim is to motivate and empower you to overcome the different elements that characterize your social anxiety.

3 We approach your social anxiety and shyness as unique and specific issues that may be very different from other people's experiences. You will see, from some of the many examples we quote in this book, that social anxiety affects people in many different ways; we tailor the solutions to your unique situation. We are not exponents of a 'one-size-fits-all' approach to treating shyness. Also, we avoid discussing the all-too-obvious example of public speaking being the main context in which this kind of anxiety most presents. Before introducing skills and ideas for overcoming social anxiety when we work with people professionally, we first listen very carefully to their experiences and stories about their difficulty. Of course, it is impossible to 'listen' to a personal story in a book. However, we reflect in this book the diverse contexts and struggles that we encounter with our clients, in order to convey the complex nature of the difficulty and allow you to begin to understand and overcome your own social anxiety.

4 The primary focus of the book is on psychological skills and techniques that you can apply to overcoming your social anxiety or shyness. These skills are derived from the findings of modern psychological research. The focus will be on what you can *do* and how you can *think* about situations differently so as to help you on your way. You will be able to see and measure your progress at each step of the way. You may be relieved to know that this process will not start with questions about your childhood, even though your earlier years may have some vague reference to your social anxiety. Modern psychological approaches focus on what is happening to you now and what you can do to bring about change, rather than on developing deep insight into your situation. You may find that some of the ideas you come across in the book can even be used and applied to help you in other areas of your life which present a challenge for you. We base our ideas not only on tried and tested clinical experience, but also on modern psychological approaches such as Cognitive Behavioural Therapy and family-systems therapy. We are interested in how people experience embarrassment or shame and how these, in turn, affect how they relate to those around them. We find that there is a circular relationship between shame and social anxiety. We will say more about this later on in the book.

This is an extensive and practical self-help book derived from modern evidence-based clinical practice. It is designed to help you, the shy or socially anxious person (or a person who is affected by or related to someone with shyness or social anxiety), to gain confidence and the proven techniques and skills needed to overcome the fear. The book will engage you in reflection and will encourage you to try out new skills and tasks. It will help you to develop an understanding of your own way of thinking about social anxiety and enable you to select and try out the psychological techniques that are likely to help you. At various points in each chapter you will find 'Stop and think' exercises (see pages 6–7), which are designed to help you apply the information and techniques to your own situation.

As a point of distinction from some other methods and books on social anxiety, we have tried to avoid presenting a fixed 'menu' of ways to reduce anxiety. The main emphasis is on helping you, the reader, to acquire a comprehensive clinical and psychological understanding of shyness and its resolution. This improves the likelihood of successfully reducing anxiety and increases your active engagement in the relevant issues. The book is structured so that you will be empowered to confront the general, as well as the more unique and idiosyncratic, characteristics of your social anxiety.

We sometimes meet people in clinical settings who find that taking the step to get counselling for social anxiety has been too big a challenge and who do not quickly get the results they wanted. If the behaviour which you are targeting to try to change has not shifted, in spite of your efforts or having worked through this book, it is worth re-examining the nature of your difficulties once again, rather than concluding that there must be something more serious or untreatable about you! This is unlikely to be the case, and therefore we would encourage readers who do not feel that they have made progress in the past to take a fresh look at what they are experiencing. There may be several reasons why success has not come in the way you had hoped. Here are some possible reasons:

- Without individual preparation and assessment, it can be difficult to identify the techniques which are most likely to work for your own social anxiety.
- You may be trying to use too many of the techniques that you have come to understand, or not selecting those which are most appropriate for you.
- If you have attended a group for social anxiety, it may be that some of the techniques most likely to work for you have not been included in that course.
- For some people, they may have been given too much information about the nature of their shyness, which may inadvertently have increased their anxiety.
- Your difficulty with shyness and social anxiety may be being 'driven' by another issue, and this may need to be identified and treated in the first instance.
- It is possible that you may not be experiencing classic social anxiety, or that the sense of shame or embarrassment you experience has not been fully addressed. An effect of this may be that

some of the skills and techniques you have learned may not work for you yet.

Some people who experience shyness or social anxiety prefer to work with a counsellor, therapist or psychologist to help them achieve their goals. If this is the case for you, this book may be a useful companion in that context. For a few readers, taking the step to contact a trained professional who can help them is in itself stressful and anxiety-provoking. They may worry about how they will come across and present themselves to the helping professional, and that their greatest fear – that they will come across badly – may inhibit them from starting this process. If this is the case, we hope that some of the ideas covered in this book will help you either to take that first step to contact a trained professional, or to start some of the therapeutic journey on your own. At the end of this book, you will have an understanding of your own social anxiety and how it affects you, and you will also be able to identify the techniques which are most likely to work for you. You will then be able to concentrate on putting these into practice. It is important to undertake an individual assessment of your anxiety, rather than to assume that everyone who experiences social anxiety is alike. You can also use this book to help you practise what you have learned between sessions with your therapist.

If you are working through this book on your own or with help from a friend or relative, there are some things you can do to make the time and effort you invest in this process as rewarding as possible. A good starting point is to decide when and where you will work with this book. Chose a time and place when you will be able to read and think comfortably. You may find it useful to make regular short appointments with yourself and write these in your diary or electronic calendar. Remember that learning new skills and techniques takes regular practice, so half an hour a day for a week or two might be more effective that a two-hour 'blitz' at the weekend. You may also find it helpful to have a notebook to write in as you work through this book.

You will see that each chapter has several 'Stop and Think' exercises labelled with this symbol:

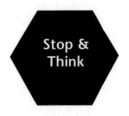

It can be very tempting to skip over these, but we would encourage you to spend some time doing the exercises. They are specifically designed to help you reflect on the material in this book and practise the techniques we describe. Use your notebook to record your reflections and practice.

As social anxiety varies so widely, no one book can cover everything that everyone needs. What we can do, though, is outline the psychological techniques that are most likely to work, and show you how to use them. Once you have been introduced to these skills, you can try them out for yourself. You may also need to use other sources of information, such as those listed in 'Useful addresses' at the end of this book.

What's in the rest of this book?

The rest of this book contains information, techniques to practise, and advice. Not all of this will be useful to everyone, but you will find guidance on how to select and try the techniques most likely to work for you. The book is almost entirely practical in its focus. It is oriented to helping you first to understand the source or cause of your social anxiety from a psychological perspective. Through case studies, it describes in detail the different presentations of shyness, helping you to recognize how your own difficulty with social anxiety affects you. It then goes on to highlight the wide variety of potential triggers which must be identified and treated in order to overcome this challenge. The final chapters cover the information, skills and techniques you will need to begin formulating your own individual treatment plan.

Throughout this book, we have shared many case studies which illustrate the way in which people we have worked with have found social situations difficult and how they have overcome their shyness or anxiety. These examples are based on real situations and people but we have changed details that might identify them or the context in which they live, in order to preserve their confidentiality.

We have tried to present a book that is written in a user-friendly and jargon-free style. A criticism sometimes levelled at psychologists is that, at times, we use and refer to concepts and terms that may not be familiar to many people. We have tried to avoid psychobabble and to focus instead on what is practical and usable. It is helpful, though, to understand a bit more about the background and causes of social anxiety if treatment is to be effective. We will aim to help this process by avoiding terms and language that may feel alienating or unfamiliar. Briefly, here is what each chapter contains:

- **Chapter 2** explores the experience of being shy, anxious or fearful about social situations. It contains a number of case studies which illustrate each individual's experience and how varied fears of social situations can be. It describes the impact that social anxiety can have on many people's lives. We discuss how common it is, the statistics, who is most affected; and what people fear the most when experiencing difficulties in social situations. We also address the common causes and symptoms of shyness and social anxiety. We discuss why there is probably no single approach to treating social anxiety which will be effective for everyone.

- **Chapter 3** helps you to understand more about how *you* experience social anxiety. We cover the range of situations that may produce social anxiety and that may also lead to different levels of intensity of the unpleasant feelings. We also discuss what physical reactions there may be to anxiety and consider the thoughts that anxious people may have that reinforce the feelings they experience. In this and later chapters in the book, we go on to show how to use this understanding to start managing your social anxiety. We include some case studies in order to illustrate the explanations that we give. Again, this chapter will show the wide range of ways in which social anxiety presents, and will assist you in mapping your individual situation as a first step to selecting the appropriate techniques which will help you.

- **Chapter 4** considers why and how your efforts to overcome shyness or social anxiety may not always succeed. This is an important point of focus, as many people who experience personal challenges in their life will have already attempted various methods or means to overcome their difficulty. If the difficulty continues, it is important and helpful to understand why the solution that you have attempted has failed. Avoidance of difficult situations is one example. If we are anxious about a particular social situation and withdraw before exposing ourselves to it, it is likely that the anxiety will persist. Avoidance is understandable, but it is unlikely to be the most effective solution. This chapter will again use case studies to explain this and help you to understand how and why your progress in overcoming shyness may be more limited that you had hoped. We also introduce the psychological approach we use clinically and in this book, Cognitive Behavioural Therapy (CBT). While we highlight many of the ideas that are currently in use in this type of therapy, we emphasize that it is a good idea to avoid a 'one-size-fits-all' approach.

- **Chapter 5** focuses on the behavioural, or 'doing', techniques that are most likely to help you to manage and overcome awkwardness, embarrassment and anxiety in social situations. We identify what you can do by way of using skills and techniques that should reduce your anxiety. The main focus of this chapter is reducing self-consciousness, which is a major contribution to shyness and social anxiety for many people. We also describe how to move from avoidance to coping in situations you may find difficult.

- **Chapter 6** describes how managing your physical reactions to anxiety using structured exercises and 'quick fix' techniques should help to improve your confidence in this area. The emphasis in this chapter is on how to reduce physical tension and some of the unpleasant sensations that we experience when we become anxious.

- **Chapter 7** takes the thinking further and examines what drives or reinforces shyness and social anxiety. The major driving factor is often the way in which we come to think about what happens when we encounter others in social situations. Common themes include being hypercritical of your performance or anxiously monitoring how other people respond to you. This chapter will explain this, in straightforward language, and help you to identify ways in which thinking can drive or reinforce your anxiety.

- **Chapter 8** takes this further with some helpful suggestions on how changing the way you think may help with your social anxiety. For example, reframing anxious thoughts is an effective way of reducing anxiety. A particular focus is how we respond to and manage experiences such as blushing or stammering. This chapter uses case studies and coaching tips to support you in using CBT tools to reframe anxious thoughts.

- **Chapter 9** has a slightly different emphasis in that it is oriented towards supporting a friend or relative who may have difficulties with shyness or social anxiety. We offer ideas and guidance on how to help others who are affected in this way. This chapter will also show friends and relatives how to support others who become anxious in social situations in using the techniques that they have learned in this book. This chapter is especially important as social anxiety is, by its nature, a source of disruption to social interaction and relationships. Therefore, if we acquire skills and confidence in helping others to manage their anxiety, this can help them to take the necessary steps to confront their fears and gain experience in social situations which will help them to overcome their shyness.

- **Chapter 10** is oriented towards readers who find that self-help may not be enough. For readers who still find themselves unacceptably anxious in social situations, this chapter will help you to realize that what you have learned from reading the book is a necessary, and possibly first, step towards overcoming the difficulty. We also point out that some people with social anxiety may require the aid of a qualified counsellor, psychotherapist or psychologist to help them with certain aspects of the challenge they face. Seeking the help and support of a suitably qualified professional is a further proactive and positive step that you can take in order to overcome the difficulty. The chapter will explain how to find a suitably qualified person to work with, and what you might expect from sessions with him or her.

The ideas presented in this book are based on tried and tested methods. They come from the experience that we and many colleagues use to help treat people with social anxiety. The book is not full of theory and textbook ideas. It is, rather, a companion text to help you understand and address your difficulties. We wish you luck in taking the first step to try and overcome social anxiety, and we hope that you enjoy working through the book. You have already made the move towards trying to understand your fear and working to overcome it. This motivation can only help to bring you probable success in return for your hard work.

2

What are shyness and social anxiety?

We have written this book in order to bring together the knowledge and skills which are likely to be useful for anyone who struggles when encountering situations, events or places which involve interacting with other people. We know that for a very few people almost every social event is frightening and something to be avoided. A much larger proportion of people might describe themselves as shy, nervous or awkward around other people. This type of difficulty may be limited to a particular group of people, for example colleagues rather than friends; to a specific activity, such as asking for a refund in a shop; or to events such as parties or team meetings at work. If you are shy or socially anxious, you will know that the physical sensations, emotions and thoughts that occur in the situations you find difficult are unpleasant and uncomfortable.

Terms such as 'shyness', 'social anxiety' and 'social phobia' refer to similar difficulties and are often used interchangeably. In this book we generally refer to 'shyness' and 'social anxiety', so what are we talking about? For the purposes of this book, they are anxious or fearful reactions to situations or events in a social context (i.e. involving other people) which have a noticeable effect on a person's life. We occasionally use the term 'social phobia' to refer to social anxiety which has a particularly marked negative impact on a person's life.

Essentially, social anxiety is what the name implies – anxiety provoked by social situations. Shyness is very much the same difficulty – feeling anxious, awkward or embarrassed in social situations. Many people think of social anxiety as a 'clinical' or more disabling form of shyness. Our experience has shown us that people who refer to their difficulties as social anxiety, social phobia or shyness all struggle with very similar issues. They also encounter overlapping or similar negative effects on their personal, family and professional lives. We have come to believe that the terms are largely interchangeable and that the important thing is to understand and work with your unique challenges.

Books and research that discuss social anxiety often describe people who find it difficult to give speeches or presentations in public, or to interact with groups of people they don't know very well. Our experience has shown us that, while social anxiety does make it very difficult for some people to speak in public, there are many other ways in which it may present. Here are some examples of people with whom we have worked:

Jane went to a school near her home in the country where there were never more than 20 students in her class and there were strict rules about being silent unless selected to answer a question in lessons. When she went to university, some of her lectures were attended by over 100 noisy students who would mutter comments throughout the sessions. She became very anxious in lectures and began to avoid them, borrowing notes from friends to catch up.

Richard was simply described as 'the shy one' by his family. As a young child, he had always seemed more interested in playing on his own than with other children at school or at home. His teachers appreciated having at least one member of the class who needed little encouragement to get on with his own work, and Richard did well at university, although he seldom joined in clubs or activities there. When he graduated, Richard went to work running the 'back office' of the family business but his parents worried about his increasing isolation.

Sahir came to England as a young adult to stay with his cousins, who had been born here. He found their terraced house in a friendly neighbourhood very different from the small quiet town in the Middle East where he had grown up. He found his new English neighbours loud and slightly frightening and became very anxious talking to anyone except his cousins.

Geoff loved his job as an electrical engineer and was often the centre of lively technical discussions at work which frequently kept projects on track or saved time or money. Away from work, however, he felt awkward and ill at ease in conversations and would almost never agree to go to parties or other social events. When he did, he would feel himself stammer, blush and begin to feel nauseous, and would almost always go home early.

Ellie taught her science classes in secondary school with confidence and was admired by her colleagues for her ability to keep the most challenging groups of teenagers under control. She dreaded parents' evenings though, shaking and sweating when she tried to hold conversations with her students' parents.

Jane, Richard, Sahir, Geoff and Ellie all struggled with a form of social anxiety, which many of their friends and family called shyness. Their stories and the situations which triggered their anxiety are, however, very different. The common theme is that their anxiety was provoked by specific situations which involved other people – large groups of students for Jane, noisy but friendly English neighbours for Sahir, and so on. They also reacted in very different ways. We will encourage you to think about your unique difficulties later. For now, we hope that you are beginning to see that social anxiety is more than just a fear of public speaking. It encompasses a wide range of anxious reactions to a large variety of social situations. This is why a 'one–size-fits-all' solution is unlikely to work. Each individual who struggles with shyness or social anxiety has unique difficulties which are best overcome, or at least managed, using techniques tailored to that person's particular situation.

What do we mean by social situations?

In a nutshell, a social situation is any situation, event, party, gathering or encounter with other people. It might be a conversation with one other person, a small group of parents meeting in a playground, a large team meeting at work, a party or a big event such as a concert. Most people who seek help for social anxiety find that their anxiety is provoked by a specific set of circumstances. They might, for example, feel confident among a group of friends but struggle to take part in team meetings at work. Or perhaps they can deal confidently with small groups but not large ones. Alternatively they might feel happier when they can 'lose themselves' in a crowd than in smaller groups where others may pay more attention to them.

You almost certainly encounter a variety of social situations every day. Using public transport, visiting the dentist or doctor, going to school or work – all these are social situations. Other examples include shopping, parties, family holidays and so on. Most people we work with can manage some social situations more easily than others, and we will encourage you to think about what you can already do well. Later chapters in the book will show you how to tackle the situations which you personally find particularly challenging.

What is an anxious reaction?

Our minds and bodies are designed to keep us safe from danger, and the features which do this have evolved over thousands of years. While they are often very good at keeping us safe, unfortunately some aspects of the way in which this works are more appropriate for life in ancient or prehistoric times rather than the Western world in the twenty-first century.

In dangerous situations, our mind quickly identifies the threat and, as you may know, causes the production of adrenaline, which floods into our circulation. This prepares our body to react by defending ourselves, running away or standing very still – the 'fight, flight or freeze' response. Because this needs us to be able to use lots of energy quickly, our heart rate and blood pressure increase, our digestive system slows down and we become physically tense. All these physical sensations are unpleasant and uncomfortable: we may feel hot and sweaty, faint, dizzy, nauseous or have a headache. They are side effects of our instinctive attempts to be safe.

While it may seem strange, we have evolved to react in this way to situations which threaten our part in social groups. Thousands of years ago, it was vital to survival to be part of groups such as tribes or families. Isolated individuals were unlikely to survive, so our ancient ancestors evolved a strong drive to succeed at maintaining good social connections. This meant that their tribe or family would offer protection in dangerous situations. Any social situation which became awkward, tense or embarrassing threatened that safety and would provoke anxiety. At that time, social anxiety was a useful tool: it encouraged people to make and maintain the social bonds which kept them safe from enemies and predators. Although in modern society it is theoretically possible – if not generally an enjoyable way to live – to survive safely in isolation, we are still 'tuned' to react in this way to social situations which we think of as challenging and which threaten to leave us isolated or shamed.

Fear is the normal response to perceived danger or stress, although like many types of anxiety a fear of social situations is often not helpful, as we will explain. It becomes a psychological difficulty when it is out of proportion, prevents us from doing things which we can achieve or goes on for too long. For a few, it may be linked to traumatic experiences such as being teased, rejected or bullied, while others of us may have experienced difficulties during a particular stage of our lives, for example when starting school or leaving home to live apart from family.

Once we experience shyness, the way in which our body reacts to the situations we fear may dramatically make the situation worse for us. These reactions may include stammering, blushing, hunching our bodies forward or speaking with a low-pitched tone of voice, as well as other changes in the way we think, feel and behave. Changes in the way we speak or move are often driven by a desire to feel safe. Unless these changes are managed, we may have the sensation of 'spinning out of control', causing increased fear, discomfort and anxiety. We may then worry about other people noticing our anxiety and we become increasingly self-conscious and preoccupied with the unpleasant effects and symptoms of fear. Unfortunately these mutually reinforce one another, and this can lead us to avoid social situations completely. When this occurs, there is often a sense of hopelessness which leads us to wonder: 'Will I ever overcome my difficulties?' Despite the doubt, the majority of people who engage in therapy have successfully managed to beat their fear.

Blushing

Many people tell us that they find blushing especially distressing. This may be particularly acute if you are shy, because you are likely to think that your symptoms are obvious and shameful to everyone around you. As we will explain later, as therapists our approach to symptoms like this is twofold: reducing self-consciousness and learning relaxation will help manage the physical sensations, and working with the way you think about these symptoms and what other people think will reduce your anxiety.

Blushing is the visible effect of increased blood flow to small blood vessels near the skin. It most often occurs on the face, neck and chest, although it can happen anywhere on the body, and may be accompanied by excessive sweating. This increased blood flow is an automatic reaction of our nervous system and not something we can consciously control. While it is often the result of feeling anxious or embarrassed, it can also be caused by some medication or certain medical conditions. If it is having a significant effect on your life, it is important to check possible causes with your GP.

If your blushing is a response to shyness or anxiety, you may consider it to be one of the most important aspects of your difficulty to manage. Because we cannot consciously control the automatic physical processes which result in blushing, the only way to reduce its impact is to work on reducing the anxiety you feel. For most people this requires a combination of the doing and thinking techniques we describe later. This may seem an indirect approach, but our experience and significant amounts of research show that it is often effective. You might find it useful to think of blushing as the way in which you measure your progress in coping with shyness. As you work through this book and your coping improves, we hope that your blushing will reduce. If that isn't happening, it may indicate that you need to select other techniques to target your unique difficulties.

The experience of social anxiety, social phobia and shyness

Everyone experiences fear and anxiety at some time in their lives; these are normal reactions to certain situations, although they may differ between people and situations. In fact, anxiety is useful and at times potentially life-preserving, so it could be argued that it might be dangerous if we did not experience some anxiety in certain circumstances. Anxiety helps sends messages to the brain that rapidly prompt us to escape from threatening situations, such as an encounter with a dangerous animal or a threatening or abusive person. Almost everyone experiences some anxiety before doing something for the first time or when we fear we could let ourselves down. This might be going on a first date, having to give a speech at work or at a wedding, when sitting down to an exam or attending a job interview or many other situations. Some anxiety, psychologists have argued, helps us to perform better than if we had no anxiety at all. Too much anxiety or anxiety that carries on for a long time, however, may become overwhelming and can interfere with our ability to cope or to perform. This is true of social anxiety: some anxiety during social situations is normal and in fact very common; too much worry about doing something that could result in embarrassment or humiliation before, during and after social contact may affect your enjoyment and pleasure, as well as your ability to cope with a range of social experiences. Of course, some people feel so overwhelmed by their anxiety that they choose to avoid all situations where they may encounter the unpleasant effects of it. That is why so many people who have social anxiety will either avoid or reduce the possibility of social contact whenever they possibly can, sometimes making excuses, bowing out of invitations or developing stories to get out of stress-producing situations. Others continue to socialize whenever they can, but they never really feel at ease because their thoughts and actions are somehow maintaining their fears of social situations. In order to understand more about how social anxiety might affect you, we need to look at how people are affected generally by anxiety, fears and phobias. Since social anxiety is a form of anxiety, this understanding helps us to gain insight into what we may feel when we start to think about social situations.

What are the implications of being shy or socially anxious?

Being shy or socially anxious may have significant negative effects on an individual's personal, family or professional life. We know that the impact is not limited to the individual affected: partners, family, friends and colleagues may all be affected as well.

In our personal lives, being shy or socially anxious may have a range of effects. It could mean that we simply don't enjoy social occasions or parties as much as we would like because we do not feel that we 'join in' as much as everyone else. For those who are moderately shy it may even mean that they miss out on many such occasions because they feel too awkward to attend. If you find social situations challenging, it may be difficult to form good friendships or intimate relationships. Shyness or social anxiety can be a major factor in difficulties with self-esteem or confidence.

> Richard, whom we described earlier in this chapter, is an example. After leaving university, he had few friends and rarely went out, preferring to spend his evenings at home. He would tell his parents that he didn't think he had the ability to make friends, saying that he had just never learnt how to do it.

Many people who have this type of difficulty describe the impact it has on their family life. This may be because it becomes hard to take part in family gatherings, holidays, activities with children and so on. It may be that these situations are simply more stressful and less enjoyable than they might be, or that the whole family is affected because the family member concerned tends to avoid taking part. This in turn can put relationships under strain and have a negative impact on children's development.

> *Brenda* had always felt she was the 'odd one out' among her noisy and outgoing family. As an adult she tended to avoid family gatherings, making up various excuses for her absence. When her husband's parents invited a large number of guests to their fortieth wedding anniversary party, Brenda refused to go, saying that she just couldn't cope with large groups of people. Her husband was so hurt by this that he walked out of the family home and threatened to divorce her if she didn't 'sort herself out'.

Careers and professional achievement can be severely limited by difficulties in coping with social situations. Very few jobs involve working in complete isolation: almost all demand some form of interaction with colleagues, teams and managers. People who are shy or socially anxious often find that they are limited in the careers they can comfortably follow or the success they achieve.

Not taking a regular active part in team meetings, for example, might have a negative effect on your annual appraisal or prospects for promotion. Ellie's struggle with aspects of her role as a teacher, described on p. 14, shows just how great an impact such difficulties can have.

Who experiences social anxiety?

The simple answer to this question is 'almost anybody'! Recent research suggests that up to half the adult population will describe themselves as chronically shy and another 10 to 15 per cent will describe themselves as shy in at least one specific situation. Indeed, one published survey reported that only 5 per cent of adults do not consider themselves to be shy. Up to 8 per cent of the adult population may meet the more stringent formal criteria for a diagnosis of social phobia.

There is no extensive research which can identify particular cultural backgrounds, socio-economic groups or demographic characteristics which are more likely to be associated with higher rates of shyness or social anxiety. Some older research reported higher rates of shyness among women when compared with men, but more recent reports do not show a significant difference. This may be because it has recently become more acceptable for men to describe themselves as shy or admit to difficulties related to shyness or social anxiety.

How do people become anxious in social situations?

There are many reasons why people may become shy, awkward or anxious in social situations. For each individual, it is likely that there is more than one factor which contributes to your anxiety and these will combine in a way that is unique to you. Here are some of the more common factors that may play a part in this type of difficulty:

- *Inherited or genetic factors* Some of every individual's psychological and emotional characteristics are determined by their genetic makeup at birth. Some of these inherited characteristics may mean that we are predisposed to become shy or anxious in social situations. Stammering, for example, may sometimes be a product of our genetic makeup and will understandably make us more likely to be shy. While we cannot change this, it is possible to learn effective ways of coping with inherited characteristics.

- *Learned behaviour* Whatever characteristics we might have inherited, there are many aspects of how we feel, what we think and what we do which we learn from experience, whether as a child or an adult. We might, for example, have become anxious at large family gatherings as children, perhaps because they can be noisy or because relatives made silly or embarrassing comments such as 'Oh, haven't you grown!' This could translate to being anxious in similar situations later on. As an adult, embarrassing experiences – where we think we have made a mistake in a work meeting, for example – may make us anxious in such situations in future.

- *Bullying or teasing* Adults or children become anxious when they experience reactions such as bullying or teasing which exclude them from the main group of people around them. The result can be that you become anxious around people. In effect, this experience teaches you to expect to be embarrassed, ashamed or hurt when you encounter people who behave that way, and it is understandable that that would make anyone shy, anxious or even frightened.

- *Early experiences* We learn many of our attitudes towards and skills in interacting with other people as fairly young children. If you lived somewhere isolated or your family tended not to socialize, you may not have had much opportunity to practise these skills in a way that felt safe, and this may contribute to the anxiety you feel now. If, for example, your family were particularly protective when you were young and wanted you to stay close, you may have learnt to be anxious about new people or new situations. The experience of abuse may also leave you shy or socially anxious. If this applies to you, your experiences may have other implications for your psychological wellbeing. While the techniques in this book may be helpful in improving your confidence in social situations, you may find that you would like to seek further support. Your GP or other health professionals will be able to help.

- *Being or feeling different* If you look or feel different from most of the people around you, this may contribute to you becoming anxious when you have to interact with those people. This might happen, for example, if you are disabled in some way or have moved to a new country and live in an area where there are few people who share your physical characteristics or cultural background. It could also be the case that you simply do not share the same interests as the groups of people who make you anxious. If you were interested in gardening but not science fiction on television, for example, you would expect to feel awkward, out of place and probably anxious at a *Star Trek* convention!

- *Other psychological factors* The experience of stress, low mood, anxiety and many other mental health issues can make it more difficult to interact with people, and this in turn may make you more prone to being shy or socially anxious. If this is a significant factor for you, you may find that you do not make the progress you would like using the skills in this book until you address other psychological factors first. Depression, for example, often results in people withdrawing from social situations, and it may be that working on that low mood is the most helpful way to improve confidence in social situations. If this is the case for you, we would strongly recommend that you talk to your GP or a mental health professional.

- *Medication* Some prescribed medication is associated with an increase in feelings of anxiety generally. This may have an impact on confidence in social situations and increase feelings of shyness or discomfort. If you think this might apply to you, talk to your GP or other health professional.

You may be able to make an assessment of how you have become shy or anxious by reflecting on the list above. As we describe later, it is not always necessary to have a complete and comprehensive explanation of how your difficulties may have arisen in order to begin overcoming them. It is, however, often useful or reassuring to understand how your individual characteristics and background may have contributed to your current anxiety or shyness. If you would like more help in understanding this aspect of yourself, it may be useful to consult a psychologist or other mental health professional.

What would it be like if I successfully managed my shyness?

Working through a self-help book or engaging with a therapist or counsellor is a commitment, so it is important to be clear about why you are investing this time and effort. If you are reading this because you struggle in a particular set of social situations, you can probably identify the issue. It is equally important, however, to keep in mind what it might be like to successfully manage your difficulties. Each individual we have worked with is so different that it is impossible to give a general description of what it might be like to manage or overcome your shyness, but here are some ideas that might encourage you to persevere.

- Coping with shyness may mean that you can start to enjoy activities or occasions with family and friends which you previously dreaded.
- Reducing your anxiety may support your work by making it less stressful or even making it possible to move to roles you once thought were too challenging.
- Relationships which have been put under strain by your anxiety may improve.
- Your general mental health may improve as your confidence increases.
- Your physical health may improve as you become less anxious.

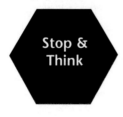

Stop & Think

Why are you reading this book? What do you want to achieve? What aspects of your life would improve if you were able to manage your shyness? Even if you were still somewhat shy, what would it be like to improve your ability to manage social situations?

How can I overcome my social anxiety?

Of course, we would say, 'Start by reading this book', so you have already taken a very positive step! As we said before, shyness and social anxiety are very treatable psychological difficulties and there are skills and techniques you can learn yourself which are likely to be effective in overcoming your anxiety. This book will take you through the following stages:

- helping you to understand your individual difficulties in different social situations;
- helping you to look at why the ways in which you have tried to overcome your anxiety may not have worked as you would like;
- teaching you the techniques most likely to help you overcome your anxiety;
- describing how to find further sources of help if you need more support than a book can deliver.

The basis of the understanding, skills and techniques we teach in this book is Cognitive Behavioural Therapy (CBT). This approach is well established and has been shown by extensive research to be effective in managing and reducing anxiety – so much so that it is the main approach recommended by the National Institute for Health and Clinical Excellence (NICE) in the UK, which evaluates treatments for use in the NHS. The term 'Cognitive Behavioural Therapy' describes this way of working quite well: the focus is on what you think (cognitive) and what you do (behavioural). That is why the later chapters in this book concentrate on techniques that work with how you think and what you do.

The most important thing to remember for now is that overcoming your difficulties will require time, effort and patience. Unfortunately there is no 'magic wand' which will reduce your anxiety overnight. The good news is, however, that there are proven and effective techniques which you can learn.

Think back to the last time you learnt a new skill; you might remember learning to drive, or ride a bicycle, or even how to use your latest mobile phone. Almost certainly, you needed to build that skill in small steps and had to do quite a lot of practice before you became confident in your abilities. Learning the skills in this book will be similar to those experiences. That means you are most likely to get the greatest benefit if you set aside short periods of time frequently to work through this book a section at a time, rather than reading it all at one sitting. Half an hour, two or three times a week over several weeks, is more likely to be effective than trying to cover everything in one long session. The many 'Stop and Think' exercises throughout this book help you work this way, because they are designed to encourage you to take the time to think about what you have read and apply it to your own unique difficulties. In this way, you are most likely to make progress and to learn the skills you need.

When we are learning anything, from school subjects such as history or physics to skills such as riding a bicycle or managing shyness, it is important to have the time and space to do that. Most of us have busy lives with multiple demands from family, friends, jobs and the like, and time to invest in yourself can be difficult to find. It can also often feel very selfish to spend time on ourselves when there are so many demands on that time. With the sort of work we describe in this book, however, other people are likely to benefit as you become less shy and more able to join them in the activities you find difficult. Depending on your own circumstances, it may be useful to explain to friends or family that you are taking positive steps to improve your skills in social situations, and that this means you need some 'study time' in order to do this. Many people also find it useful to make an appointment with themselves for the times when they will work on these skills, and write it in their diary or calendar. Find a place to study, ideally fairly quiet and free of distractions, and let people know that, just for the short time you will be working, you would like to be left to concentrate. Use your notebook for jotting down ideas as you read and for doing the 'Stop and think' exercises. Here is the first one:

Stop & Think

Where and when are you likely to be able to work on developing the skills we describe in this book? Try making two or three short appointments with yourself for the next week. Do you need to ask anyone else to help keep that time free of distraction? For example, would your partner or a friend watch the children or answer the phone for you? Do you have a notebook you can use so that all your notes stay together? Plan a small reward for yourself after each study session. This might be a simple as a soak in the bath or a walk – anything you enjoy.

3

Understanding my shyness

Everyone feels anxious in some social situations, but pervasive and more persistent forms of this, such as blushing, stammering and shyness, can provoke distressing feelings of fear of these situations. People with social anxiety react to feelings, experiences, places or events involving contact with people as if they were a danger or a threat. This can be very difficult for both the individual and others, because it makes everyday situations uncomfortable and it restricts and interferes with people's lives. Research shows that it is often our response to anxiety that keeps it going. So even if you do not know how your social anxiety first began, you can still learn to control or overcome it by gradually changing your responses in social situations. If you have always been shy or had difficulty with making friends, it may be time to look at your individual coping cycle to really understand how it affects you. This chapter illustrates some of the ways in which social anxiety presents, and helps you to map your individual situation as a first step to selecting various techniques that will gradually help you conquer your fear.

Social anxiety is a specific type of anxiety difficulty. Anxiety affects your body, your thoughts and your actions and reactions. It is mostly accompanied by a sense that something unpleasant or bad is about to happen. You may think that you will do something embarrassing or humiliating when interacting with other people, either in person, on the phone or via the computer, so that they will judge you or think that you are in some way inferior, odd, different, stupid, strange or not worthy of their attention.

> I was fine until I had to speak. They all focused their attention on me and I felt a jolt in my stomach. Here we go . . . I can feel my face growing hotter and redder by the minute, the words get stuck in my throat and

all I seem to be able to manage is a silent whisper: 'Hello – my name is Jonathan.' The vice-president looks at me and says, 'Welcome to our team, Jonathan.' Again, there is silence . . . people are waiting for me to say something. I can feel my heart beating faster, my knees are trembling . . . My thoughts are racing. Can they see how anxious I am? Have they noticed that I am shaking? Does my voice sound strange? I finally manage to clear my throat and I start speaking. At first my voice is low and my sentences are short – surely they must think I am an idiot. How could I ever do my job and manage other people if I can't actually introduce myself to a small group of people on my first day at work? They might as well sack me now because there is no way that I can handle this team . . . or for that matter any other human beings . . . because I am petrified of people. I feel so ridiculous that I ask for a glass of water to make out that I have a sore throat. This works: the vice-president starts talking again, giving the rest of the team a talk on how brilliant I am. I sigh with relief but only because I do not have to talk . . . or at least not for now. I cringe and look away. These people are perhaps being fooled for now but with time they will come to learn how utterly useless and stupid I really am. I feel like a fraud.

(Jonathan, aged 40)

Jonathan's story illustrates common doubts and fears that are likely to escalate during social interactions: fear of making a fool of oneself, fear of being humiliated, fear of being evaluated by others in a negative way, fear of not fitting in, fear of attracting unwanted attention to oneself, fear of not being good enough or somehow disappointing others. It is Jonathan's fears that lead him to act in a certain way – focusing his attention too much on his inner experiences, being too self-critical, pretending to have a sore throat to avoid introducing himself to the group and assuming that he knows how other people think of him.

But despite feeling uncomfortable before and during the initial meeting with his new team, Jonathan was able to start his new job. This brought him a step closer to managing his fear. When he first sought help from a psychologist he had avoided teamwork for the previous six years, after having experienced a difficult relationship with his manager, who would often bully him in front of colleagues. Since then, he has gradually managed to build up his confidence by working for smaller companies with a reputation of being respectful and friendly towards staff. Jonathan's next challenge is to continue to meet his colleagues and clients over the next week so that he can get to know his new work environment.

Helpful and unhelpful forms of anxiety

Imagine that you are crossing the road when all of a sudden a car hits the curb when turning the corner, causing the driver to lose control. There is a good reason to be afraid. This is helpful anxiety because there is an actual threat of injury or serious damage to one's life. Once fear is generated, the brain automatically signals for adrenaline to be released into the body, which activates our general arousal system. This biological process ensures physical arousal that helps the body to prepare for dealing with threatening situations. The main effect is to increase our heart rate so that blood can be rapidly pumped to the muscles that can help us to escape, mainly to our legs and arms. When the fear is intense enough, our animal-like instincts take over. This will often cause a person to respond in one of three ways, known as the fight–flight–freeze responses to critical events, or a combination of these. When this is active, we will want to either protect ourselves (fight), run away (flight) or remain very still so that whatever we are afraid of doesn't see us (freeze).

It is easy to see how the flight response may be crucial for escaping from the threat of being hit by a speeding car. Equally plausible is the idea that the driver may avoid hitting the pedestrian by actively fighting to regain control of the car. What may be less obvious is the way in which the freeze response is just as basic. The sound of the car hitting the curb may cause you to become temporarily immobilized. Your legs may feel as if they are glued to the pavement and you are unable to move in either direction. This may actually alert the driver to your exact presence, thereby making it easier for him or her to manoeuvre the car away from you. Fear is a healthy response to danger that can be crucial for human (and animal) survival.

If you are worried about being hit by a car every time you cross the road, however, whether or not cars are in sight, your anxious or fearful reactions to trying to cross the road have become excessive and unhelpful. While your previous experiences (such as nearly being run over crossing the road last week) will understandably make you very careful, not crossing the road may have major implications for your life. This is an example of reaching the point where feeling anxious or fearful, although understandable, becomes unhelpful. You may be using a lot of energy and time worrying about what *might* – but not necessarily *will* – happen. This is not to say that there are no risks involved in crossing the road. In fact, there is some risk involved in everything we do, whether it is gardening or travelling on the bus to work. But difficulties can arise when the probability of danger attached to any given situation is unnecessarily overestimated. This can cause us to become increasingly fearful, to the extent that we start to avoid doing the things we wish to do. This happened to Sarah, who decided to resign from work because of her fear:

> *Sarah* worked as a bank manager in the city and had been using public transport for ten years. Over the past six months, however, Sarah had become increasingly anxious during her travels to and from work. Her symptoms included dizziness, sweating, tension and sleep difficulties. She began to call in sick at work, thinking that she just needed some time away from the pressure of working in the banking industry. This made her worries even worse, as she would spend a great deal of time contemplating how intimidated she felt when surrounded by strangers on the train and the various ways she could attract unwanted attention to herself when standing in close proximity to another traveller. Sarah loved her job but felt that the strains of being negatively evaluated by fellow commuters were too difficult to bear. She eventually resigned from her job in the city and began working for a local charity.

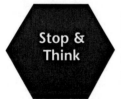

Stop & Think

As you read Sarah's story, could you see how her anxiety became unhelpful? What about your own anxiety – which aspects of it do you think are helpful and which are unhelpful?

Physical or bodily signs of anxiety

Most people who have social anxiety recognize the unpleasant physical signs of 'stress', 'worry', 'anxiety' or 'nerves'. Just experiencing them can also make you feel upset, frightened or even desperate. Some of the physical signs of anxiety can mimic physical or mental illness, which can be all the more frightening and makes things feel even worse. Psychologists who help to treat people with fears and anxiety recognize that the physical symptoms can trigger an increase in fear, which only makes the symptoms worse. This is what happens when people experience a panic attack. The physical or bodily signs that are associated with fear generally, and with a fear of social situations in particular, include the following:

- Sweating, clammy hands
- Shakiness, especially in the hands and legs
- Red rash-like patches in the face and neck area (blushing)
- Pounding heart
- Dry mouth, difficulty swallowing
- Feeling dizzy or faint
- Nausea, feeling ill, bowel discomfort or an urgent need to visit the toilet
- Headache, muscle aches and pains
- Feeling tired

Prolonged anxiety states can also affect a person's physical health. Certain physical health issues may be related to psychological difficulties, and these are termed 'psychosomatic'. The most common psychosomatic symptoms associated with social anxiety are inexplicable sweating, shivering or trembling, blushing, breathing difficulties and nauseous feelings. These conditions can be managed by treating both the symptoms and the underlying anxiety.

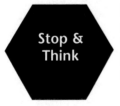
Stop & Think

How does your body react when you are shy or anxious? What do you notice most? What are the most unpleasant sensations for you? Take a few moments to make a note of your unique reactions.

What makes your fears and anxiety unique?

In terms of psychological difficulties, fears and anxiety are both similar to and in some ways different from other issues such as low mood (depression), stress or even having an eating disorder. Here are some ideas about what is unique and specific about experiencing social anxiety and fears:

- The effects are usually intense and in certain cases can require psychological and medical intervention in order to cope with them.
- They are often triggered by some form of social contact; the signs and symptoms can gradually appear during the lead-up to social situations and build up until they become overwhelming while socializing.
- Both the mind and the body are often affected, and this can make us feel overwhelmed which in turn increases our anxiety – this effect could produce physical symptoms such as blushing or excessive sweating, as already mentioned.

For some people, shyness and social anxiety can arise in certain situations but may not be present in others. For example, a person may be able to cope with family dinners at home, but the thought of having the family dinner in a restaurant may be too difficult to bear. Intense social anxiety typically leads to avoidance of those situations which we fear because we know that our anxiety will increase if we have to deal with them. Avoidance ultimately only makes the anxiety worse, because we quickly build up a defensive story about why we can't attend a party, go shopping or do something else that involves social contact. Life then becomes a series of rituals which are designed to make us feel safer, and it may be dominated by attempts to avoid the social situations we fear. The problem with avoidance is that it prevents exposure, which in turn can thwart us from taking the opportunity to build the confidence we need to manage our anxiety. Certain methods of coping may reflect understandable but unhealthy ways to manage anxiety, such as making excuses to bow out of social commitments or the use of excessive alcohol to help quell nerves during a work lunch, dinner party or first date. Alcohol may seem to be a useful and easily available remedy to social anxiety, but it does not help solve or overcome the difficulty. Not only does it increase the risk of developing an additional challenge such as alcohol dependency, it may also lead us to attribute our ability to socialize to the use of alcohol rather than our skills and techniques for interacting with others. Avoidance is a solution, but it is often an unhelpful one.

Below is a list of many of the possible fears that people talk about when they seek professional help to overcome their social anxiety.

- A fear of making a fool of oneself
- A fear of being humiliated or embarrassed
- A fear of being criticized or negatively evaluated by others
- A fear of being ignored or of people not paying attention to what one says because of an underlying fear of being seen as boring
- A fear that other people will notice one's anxiety
- A fear of not fitting in with others or being perceived as weird or somewhat different from other people
- A fear that what one says is perceived as not important or stupid, ugly, useless and so on
- A fear of the symptoms of fear (blushing, sweating, shaking or trembling, rapid breathing, etc.)

Understanding your own fear of social contact

One way to better understand your own social anxiety is to ask yourself whether you tend to be anxious across all social situations or whether certain people, places, feelings, experiences or events can make you feel more self-conscious. Sometimes social anxiety seems to go on and on and can become a lifelong issue. There can be a number of reasons for this. Some people may have an anxious personality or have 'learned' to worry. Others may have a series of stressful life events to cope with, for example bereavements, redundancy or divorce. Others may be under pressure at work, or at home because of family problems or financial difficulties.

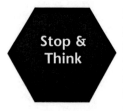

Stop & Think

How often do you feel anxious? (Often, rarely, sometimes, never.) What kinds of social situations are most likely to make you feel anxious? (Meeting new people, dealing with colleagues, eating out with friends, going on a date, talking on the phone to people, speaking to the cashier at your local bank . . .) How long does your anxiety last? (Weeks, days, hours, minutes.) Is there a pattern to your anxiety? (Does it occur on a specific day, in a specific context or place or with particular people?) How does anxiety affect you? (Eating, sleeping, concentration, memory, sex drive, energy, motivation, etc.)

People who experience social anxiety often say they are convinced other people will evaluate them in a negative way. This can make them feel vulnerable, embarrassed and ashamed. It is not uncommon for people with social anxiety to set very high standards for themselves. This can be reflected in personal assumptions such as 'I have got to do everything right to be an acceptable person' or 'I have got to look perfect at all times to ensure that other people are not disgusted or disappointed.'

Your unique experience of shyness or anxiety

It is important to recognize that each person's experience of anxiety is unique; what is perceived as 'frightening' for one person may not necessarily be the same for another. This can be reassuring in itself: no two people with social anxiety are exactly alike. This means that we might be able to ask, 'Why do other people seem to cope very well in social situations?' Now that you have reached this stage in the book, you will begin to realize that we all react to situations in very different ways. Your best friend, for example, might be very confident in social situations which make you extremely anxious. He or she might be terrified of going to the dentist, though! The manager you admire for his skill and confidence in charming new clients could be naturally this way. It is also possible that he may just be very good at concealing his anxiety. Either way, you may find it helpful later on in your work with your own difficulties to ask others for hints or even just to model your behaviour on theirs. More on this in later chapters!

A deeper understanding about the nature of anxiety and fear is useful in order to gain insight into how you think and feel before, during and after social contact. This paves the way for explaining how to overcome your social anxiety.

4

But I've tried so hard to manage my shyness – why hasn't it worked?

In the previous chapters, we described what social anxiety is and encouraged you to think about your unique challenges and difficulties. Most people who have struggled with being shy or awkward in certain social situations have tried out many solutions to these difficulties before they read a self-help book like this one or consult a therapist or psychologist. You may have attempted to reduce your shyness or anxiety using logic or common sense and been dismayed to find that these solutions have not worked. There may be many reasons for this, and it is almost certainly not that you are 'untreatable' or 'crazy'! It is much more likely that you simply have not been shown the skills and techniques most likely to help you. Another possibility is that you may have found a way of coping that worked well enough until now, which may have been ignoring the issue or avoiding challenging situations. You may also not have had the time and energy to devote to tackling these difficulties. Reading this book is a good indication that you now have the commitment, time and energy to work on overcoming your shyness.

Trying to find a solution

Since feeling anxious, awkward or shy is generally experienced as unwelcome and sometimes unpleasant, you will almost certainly have worked hard to find solutions to the way you feel and/or act in situations you find challenging. Because it is rare to have been taught about the psychological perspectives on social anxiety that we highlight in this book, most people will naturally try solutions to their difficulties based on common sense and logic. For some people, these can work well. However, it is also possible that a solution based on logic or common sense may actually help maintain your difficulties. That might seem contradictory so we have included some case studies in this chapter to illustrate what we mean. As you read them, bear in mind the most common logical solutions which people often use to try and manage their anxiety:

- avoiding situations or people you find difficult;
- intensively rehearsing what you are going to do or say;
- constantly monitoring what you are doing, saying and feeling.

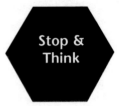

Stop & Think

Can you think how trying to solve your difficulties in these ways might either help to maintain your anxiety or have a negative effect on your personal or professional life? Here are three brief examples to illustrate what we often see working with people who ask for help with social anxiety.

Joanna enjoyed working for a small family-run firm and was worried that she would become 'just a number' when it was bought by a national chain. The owners retired and a new manager was appointed by the new company's head office. Joanna saw him deal dismissively and at times aggressively with some of her colleagues. She became anxious about meeting with or consulting him, and she became even more anxious when he complained about her absence on leave at a busy time, even though this had been agreed with the previous owners. Eventually, Joanna started to avoid him whenever possible. Unfortunately, when the new manager was moved to another branch and was asked to recommend a replacement, he put forward the name of someone from another branch. He said that Joanna had the technical skills to be a good manager but was 'too timid' to develop the necessary people skills.

John found attending formal functions with his wife, a barrister, very difficult. As a senior lecturer in theoretical chemistry, he had little in common with her colleagues and often found himself isolated in the middle of long conversations on legal strategies. In an attempt to equip himself to join in these conversations, he would spend the week before formal functions researching current legal issues in the university library and rehearsing very specific comments. He said that it often felt as if he was revising for an exam. Unfortunately, he was never able to completely predict the conversation at these functions and always felt unprepared, anxious and isolated. John would stammer and blush his way through these evenings, feeling ashamed that he could not support his wife's career by impressing her colleagues.

Fred was a London taxi driver who could make the most sullen passenger smile and was equally at ease driving in a comfortable silence. When his wife started working night shifts, he would sometimes have to go to parents' evenings at his daughter's school alone. On these occasions he would find it very difficult to talk to teachers and thought that they saw him as awkward and unintelligent. He became so focused on this that he would use all his energy during those conversations to monitor what he was saying and doing. This in turn meant that he would often not hear most of what the teachers were saying. This became such an issue that his wife persuaded him to talk to his GP, who referred him to a psychologist.

Why the first solutions we try often don't work

Joanna, John and Fred were all doing their best to solve very real difficulties using logic: Joanna avoided her difficult manager, John invested hours in preparing and Fred focused on trying to control how he felt and what he did. Unfortunately the solutions they tried all had unintended consequences or failed to reduce their anxiety: Joanna did not have the chance to learn how to approach her manager and she remained anxious, missing out on a promotion as a result. John's research often didn't prepare him for the conversation which actually took place and it increased his anxiety as he struggled to remember what he had rehearsed. Fred found that focusing inwardly on himself increased his anxiety because he constantly thought he was making mistakes. It created difficulties at home because he was never able to tell his wife what the teachers had said.

The three common logical solutions described above may not succeed in sufficiently reducing anxiety and often have unintended effects which can make the situation worse. In fact, each of them can be part of a vicious cycle which maintains anxiety. We have drawn these out in Figure 4.1.

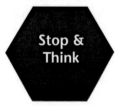

Stop & Think

How have you tried to solve your difficulties in challenging situations? Take a few minutes to note down what you have tried. Have your solutions had unintended consequences? Have they increased or reduced your anxiety?

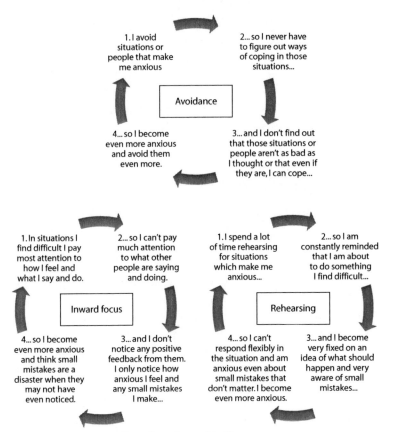

Figure 4.1 Vicious cycles of anxious thinking

Finding other solutions

So far in this chapter, we have described why some of the solutions you have worked very hard at may not have been as effective as you hoped. Rather than persisting with these solutions, the rest of this book is designed to teach you straightforward techniques based on psychological research and practice, which are known to be effective for many people with social anxiety. These techniques are designed for you to be able to practise them for yourself.

As we have already mentioned, the approach on which this book is based is Cognitive Behavioural Therapy (CBT). You may have seen reports on television about this as it is a very effective and popular psychological approach for many difficulties, particularly anxiety and depression. CBT is the approach recommended for use in treating anxiety in the UK NHS and is effective at reducing anxiety for most people. Here is a little more background on this approach.

There are three main aspects of CBT which are important to understand when working to overcome anxiety:

- The link between what we think and how we feel
- Identifying your individual response to anxiety
- Modifying solutions that have not helped

We will describe each of these in turn.

The link between what we think and how we feel

Imagine for a moment that you are fast asleep in bed at about 2.00 a.m. Suddenly you are woken by a loud noise and you think, 'There's a burglar in the house!' How would that make you feel and what would you do? You would probably feel quite scared and you might get out of bed and go somewhere safe to call for help.

Now imagine that exactly the same thing happens again and you are woken up by a loud noise. This time, however, you think, 'The cat has knocked over the laptop I left out on the kitchen table.' How would you feel and what would you do now? You might feel

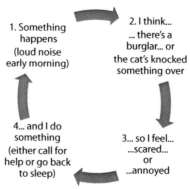

Figure 4.2 Thinking cycle

annoyed and either go back to sleep or get up to clean up the mess or shout at the cat, but you probably would not feel scared.

Can you see how two different ways of thinking about the same event have resulted in different feelings and actions? Unless you got up to investigate you wouldn't know which thought was accurate, but the way in which you think has had a large impact on what you feel and do. We have drawn this out in Figure 4.2.

This is the basis of many of the techniques in the book. Once you can identify what it is that you are thinking, you can link that to how it makes you feel. Thoughts which make you feel anxious may be valid or inaccurate. If they are not absolutely valid, the most useful techniques from this book are likely to be those which show you how to change unhelpful thoughts and alter how you feel, improving your confidence. If they are correct, the 'doing' techniques in the following chapters will help you change or manage the situation.

Identifying your individual response to anxiety

Using CBT, it is important to understand your response to anxiety in detail. A useful framework for thinking about this is to notice what you feel (your emotions), what you think, what you do and how your body feels. Here's an example:

> Ethan always became nervous at large family gatherings. Being the youngest of four children, he felt that everyone looked down on him and his job managing a local newspaper because his elder siblings all had high-profile careers in medicine or law. When his parents asked him to act as master of ceremonies for their joint retirement party, he was flattered but scared. On the point of setting out for the party, he found himself imagining various relatives commenting on his job. He even had a vivid mental picture of Uncle Jim commiserating with his parents that their youngest son was a failure. He felt frightened and ashamed and was sweating. His hands were shaking and he started to blush. He felt so bad that he rang his parents to say he was ill and stayed at home.

This description shows all four aspects of Ethan's anxious responses to a situation he found challenging. Psychologists often illustrate the way in which we respond when shy or anxious as a 'hot cross bun', as in Figure 4.3 (page 42).

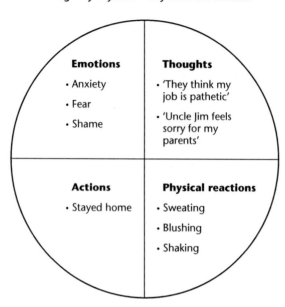

Figure 4.3 Ethan's response to anxiety – the 'hot cross bun'

The reason we are paying so much attention to your individual response to anxiety is that it helps to identify the techniques most likely to help you control your anxiety. No one can simply 'turn off' their emotions, and it would be a very dull life if we could, but we can work directly with what you think and do and how your body responds. Most people who struggle in social situations need to do all three of these, but the skills which are most likely to help you are the ones which relate to the most overwhelming part of your response to anxiety. For Ethan, his physical reactions were almost unbearable, so when he consulted a psychologist they started with relaxation techniques, such as those we describe later, to control these reactions. If the major part of your response is what you think, then you might focus on working with thoughts first. If your focus is what you do, the 'doing' techniques in this book will be useful.

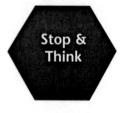

Using the notes you made about your unique social anxiety in the last chapter, can you draw your own hot cross bun? What do you think is the part of your response that you should work on first? Is it what you think or do or how your body reacts?

Modifying solutions that have not helped

The other main focus of CBT is making sure that the ways in which we try to reduce anxiety actually work. In the first part of this chapter, we talked about solutions which haven't achieved what you wanted and may even have helped to maintain your anxiety. It is crucial to your success that you monitor your progress and check that the skills and techniques you decide to try from this book actually work for you.

One way of doing this is to score your level of anxiety as you work with each technique. You might want to use a scale of 0 to 10, where 0 means you feel no anxiety and 10 means you feel as anxious as you can imagine being. Make a note of your score before you try the technique and then regularly check it as you practise the technique. Although it might take time, if your chosen solution is an effective one you should see your score reduce. If it does not do this, you may find the advice in Chapter 8 helpful. Here's an example of how this worked for Ethan when he decided to consult a psychologist who was recommended by his GP:

Ethan and his psychologist were initially struck by the overwhelming nature of his physical reactions to the anxiety provoked by family gatherings. They decided to start by working on relaxation techniques. Ethan put in a lot of practice because he was due to attend his sister's wedding three weeks after his first session with the psychologist. Over those three weeks, Ethan's score for anxiety about going to the wedding fell from 8 to 5 and he began to feel slightly more confident about joining his family there.

Unfortunately, the first person Ethan met at the wedding was Uncle Jim, who started by excitedly describing his eldest brother's promotion and then asked about Ethan's job with the local newspaper in what Ethan thought was a very condescending way. Suddenly Ethan's anxiety increased to what he later described as '11 out of 10' and he started to blush and stammer. When they talked through what had happened, Ethan and his psychologist realized that they needed to challenge the thoughts that drove Ethan's shame and anxiety before he could put the relaxation techniques into practice. With hard work, Ethan was able to go to the next family gathering – his nephew's christening, where he became a godparent and had to stand at the front of the church – with a reduced level of anxiety which only reached 3 out of 10. He was even able to get Uncle Jim laughing at tales from his newspaper!

Even working with a psychologist, counsellor or therapist, you may not start with exactly the right solution for you. The important thing is to monitor the solutions you try and only continue using them if they work for you.

Summary

Because feeling anxious is unpleasant, most people will work hard to try and reduce it. Unfortunately, the most obvious solutions often have unintended consequences and may not succeed in helping you to feel less anxious. CBT suggests other ways of working. The main focus is on challenging the way you think, if that is unhelpful, and changing what you do.

Now that you have worked through the first part of this book, you should have a good understanding of social anxiety and a clearer idea of your individual difficulties. The following chapters will develop your understanding and introduce the psychological techniques which may be more effective at reducing anxiety than the logical solutions we have described here.

5

Reducing avoidance and feelings of self-consciousness

Medication may be a useful short-term strategy for managing acute anxiety and incapacitating shyness. However, many people tell us that they would rather not use medication, particularly over long periods of time, and its use may even cause additional difficulties. The good news is that modern psychological methods are very effective in helping you overcome your fear.

A central aspect of social anxiety is feeling self-conscious. When we become very anxious, or even fearful, we tend to focus our attention inward on to ourselves so that we become painfully aware of what is happening to us. This leaves little attention for the things that are happening around us, making it difficult to hear what other people are saying or to be aware of what they are doing and how we are reacting. We have also seen that avoiding situations or people may actually maintain anxiety. Experimenting with new ways of doing things such as attending a staff party, asking more questions or making the effort to build up and maintain a social network allows you to build confidence and gradually become less anxious. This chapter describes techniques which are targeted at reducing both self-consciousness and avoidance. These are two major 'doing' techniques designed to overcome shyness. Later we move on to learning to relax as a way of managing physical symptoms of anxiety and working with anxious thoughts.

Self-consciousness and its impact on anxiety

Many aspects of social anxiety can trigger a heightened sense of self-consciousness. This includes fear of: not being accepted or of being negatively evaluated by others; feeling nervous and thinking that other people will notice and therefore think less of you; not being able to think straight; saying something that could be perceived as stupid; making a fool of yourself; blushing or stammering; and so on. Worrying about what other people think of you is likely to make you feel worse because you start to anticipate the dreaded reactions to what you may think of as your 'flaws'. A common, and seemingly logical, response to this is to focus your attention inward in an attempt to produce the very best performance you can, hiding your flaws. Unfortunately, as we illustrated earlier, when your attention is turned inwards it becomes difficult to assess what people are really saying or doing, because you may only have hazy ideas about their behaviour and reactions towards you. So in some social situations, you may know more about your inner experiences than what has actually occurred during a social encounter. Because you feel so nervous or you are convinced that you somehow will make a fool of yourself – or are sure you have already done so – you assume that other people think the same. Being self-conscious is therefore likely to increase your anxiety as you concentrate on potential mistakes and the unpleasant sensations of anxiety rather than people's reaction to you, which may be much more positive than you think.

> *David,* aged 34, was attending his cousin's birthday party. He had not been able to see his extended family much for the past year because of work. He felt nervous during the car journey over to his cousin's house, thinking that he might not have anything interesting to tell his family. After all, his life was pretty much just about work. Several thoughts were racing through his mind: what if people think I am boring, what if they ask difficult questions that I can't answer, what if they think I have turned into a weirdo? *[Worry]* When he entered his cousin's house, David felt his heart racing and he noticed that his palms were clammy *[physical symptoms of anxiety]*. Throughout the party, David kept 'checking his body' for physical signs of anxiety, feeling frightened that other people would notice that he was nervous *[overfocusing]*. He directed his attention towards the whole of his performance, constantly scrutinizing his own behaviour: am I speaking too fast, does my aunt think I am odd, can people see that I am not feeling well? The intense focus on bodily symptoms and his own performance led David to think he had made a fool of himself and that his whole family would think badly of him after the party *[interpretation]*. He muttered to himself, 'I am a social failure' *[unhelpful meanings attached to his thoughts]*. He felt increasingly uncomfortable and anxious during the rest of the party.

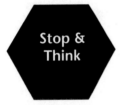

Stop & Think

Take a few moments to consider how David's inward focus on the way he felt helped to make him anxious and maintain that anxiety. The comments we have added in square brackets label the aspects of his inward focus and thinking that contributed to his anxiety.

A key aspect of overcoming your social anxiety is to learn how to reduce self-consciousness so that you can build a more balanced, and perhaps more accurate, picture of how other people view you. Learning to focus your attention on what is happening outside of yourself, instead of what is happening inside, will help you to become more engaged in social situations and feel more confident and secure about your performance.

Techniques for reducing self-consciousness

Like many of the people we have worked with, you may have put a lot of effort into the 'logical' solution of focusing on your thoughts, feelings, behaviours and physical sensations you feel in an attempt to reduce your anxiety. As we have just explained, unfortunately the most frequent result of this great effort is that you feel increasingly anxious. However, the fact that you already have a lot of practice at maintaining a specific focus can be very useful in reducing your shyness and anxiety if you can learn to direct it in a different way.

The exercises which follow are designed to help you reduce self-consciousness by focusing your attention outwards. With practice, this will reduce your anxiety. We have included several ways of doing this. You might like to start by looking through all of them and selecting the one that appeals most to work with first. Practise your selected technique until you feel confident using it when you feel relaxed. You can then move on to trying it in increasingly challenging social situations. The aim in all cases is to redirect your inward focus to what is happening around you. When you apply this in social situations, we would expect you to find that most people react positively to you most of the time. If the first technique you try isn't effective for you, we would encourage you to persevere with one of the other exercises here.

Concentration exercises

Worry is a natural way of anticipating risk and keeps us safe from catastrophe and danger. It is an automatic skill that is activated when we feel unsafe. When our perception of risk is exaggerated, we are also likely to feel unsafe and hence we start to worry to protect ourselves from the imagined fear. This is why anxious thoughts about social situations can be intense and persistent. The challenge here is to let go of your worry, because it makes you feel self-conscious and it also interferes with your ability to act, think and feel in a rational way. The concentration technique will help you to stop the flow of anxious thoughts, reduce your distress and make you feel more calm and relaxed. It will also help you to direct your attention away from your inner experiences so that you can focus on the social situation. As you begin to practise concentrating on the task in hand, try to implement the techniques in situations you regard as less threatening. You may want to start practising while alone at home before you try to reduce self-consciousness during social situations. Once you develop your ability to direct your attention away from inner experiences, you can move on to using the techniques during more challenging situations.

Listening to the lyrics of a song

Select a song that you like and then play it on your laptop, CD or music player. Concentrate on the lyrics of the song for about two minutes. Turn the playing device off and summarize the lyrics of the song out loud. Note how much of your attention is directed towards the task of listening to the song, towards yourself and towards the environment around you. You can use percentages to measure the focus of your attention. Your results might look something like this:

Concentrating on task	Yourself	The environment
50%	30%	20%

Carry out the exercise again but choose a different song. This time, concentrate on yourself – what you are thinking and feeling and the physical sensations in your body. Summarize the lyrics again and note how you divided your attention between your thoughts and sensations listening to the song and noticing the environment. This time your results might look something like this:

	Concentrating on task	Yourself	The environment
Focus on song	50%	30%	20%
Focus on you	20%	60%	20%

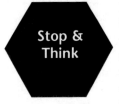

Stop & Think

Repeat the listening activities until you become adept at redirecting your attention to the task of listening to the words of the song after deliberate distraction through focusing on yourself. This will help to develop your ability to control where and when you focus your attention.

Once you are confident in paying attention to a song, practise redirecting your attention to other things – perhaps a television programme, housework, reading the paper – and eventually focusing on what someone else is saying and doing. You can then start to practise in social situations, keeping your attention on what is happening around you and what others are really doing rather than inwardly on yourself.

Paying attention to your surroundings

This exercise asks you to pay attention to the entireness of your surroundings: what you can see, feel, hear and smell. The value of this is to help you shift your focus away from inner experiences towards the more pleasant and positive aspects of your surroundings. You can use almost any situation to practise shifting your attention towards the outside world. This includes walking to your local food store, going to the park, attending a social event, visiting a museum, travelling to work or making a special meal for supper. Eventually, you can use this ability in social situations to focus on other people's genuine responses and the often pleasant aspects of the environment around you.

- Focus your attention for about six minutes on the different aspects of your surroundings.
- Now, focus your attention on what you can see (colours, objects and people).

- After about one minute begin to shift your attention towards what you can hear – the various noises around you.
- Then shift your attention to concentrate on smells before you redirect the focus towards your feelings.
- Keep moving your attention around to these different sensations. Try to vary the order of your attention to the individual sensations as this will help develop your skills in controlling your attention. Notice how you feel much more relaxed once you direct your attention away from yourself.
- Next, try to integrate your attention to include all aspects of your surroundings. Use percentages to measure the degree to which you are paying attention to each different aspect of the environment (what you can see, feel, hear and smell).

When approaching a social situation, you can use your ability to control your attention to help prevent yourself from engaging with the stream of worry that often triggers self-consciousness. Self-consciousness makes you increasingly aware of uncomfortable sensations, feelings, thoughts and behaviours. This means that you are likely to overlook important aspects of a social event such as positive cues from other people or learning interesting new things from the discussions around you. By consciously focusing on people and external aspects outside of yourself, you will feel less distressed and allow yourself to be in touch with what is happening around you. With practice you can train yourself to tune into the social world even during social situations. Below is a list of tasks you can attend to during a social event:

- Focus on what you can hear, smell and see around you.
- Listen intently to conversations or debates around you. If there is more than one conversation taking place at the same time, try to focus your attention on one of these only.
- Listen to the words the other person is saying. Shift your attention around to various people if there is more than one speaker in the group.
- Get lost in the topic. If you notice that you start to focus your attention inwards again, redirect your focus out of your head and tune into the social interaction again!

Choosing where to focus your attention

Another way of reducing the extent to which you may be focused on your internal thoughts, emotions and physical sensations is to practise using the majority of your attention in a way you choose. With practice, being able to do this in situations where you may become anxious means that you can reduce the impact that the unpleasant sensations of shyness or anxiety have on you. This does take quite a lot of practice to master but is often well worth the effort. With practice, you will be able to choose to direct your attention to the pleasant aspects of social situations – what people are talking about, the taste of good food and so on.

Start by finding a time and place where you can try this technique for a short period of time. You need to have several sounds to practise focusing on, so you may want to use a room with some external noise, such as traffic or people walking outside, and some internal sounds, perhaps a clock ticking and an electric fan.

Choose a noise in the room to focus on, the ticking clock for example, and do your best to focus on that for 20 seconds. You should find that you notice very little of the other internal noises and any external noise while you do this.

Now focus on another noise in the room for 20 seconds. You probably will not hear the first noise you focused on while you do this. Then try to focus on an external noise for 20 seconds, and you should find that you barely notice the internal sounds of the room while you are doing this.

Don't spend too long practising this skill to start with – paying attention for 20 seconds to each of three or four different sounds and then repeating that once is enough to start with. When you can confidently do this, extend the time you focus on each to 40 seconds and then to a minute.

When you are confident that you can choose where to focus your attention on your own, try the same exercise when you are with other people. You might start by practising paying attention to a close friend in a situation where you feel relaxed. When you have learnt how to do this in situations where you feel reasonably relaxed, try it in more challenging environments, choosing to pay attention to the people you are interacting with or the environment around you rather than your internal thoughts and sensations.

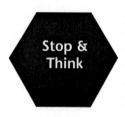

Remember that these skills take time and patience to master. Pick one that you think is most likely to work for you and try and find time to run through it at least once a day. Once you feel confident that you can control your attention in calm and quiet environments, practise in slightly noisier and more distracting places, increasing the challenge in small steps. Only move on when you are confident in each place, and keep practising until you feel confident you will be able to focus on the environment around you rather than on yourself in situations that make you feel anxious.

Reducing avoidance

We have seen that avoiding situations, events or people that trigger feelings of shyness or anxiety may not be a helpful solution to your difficulties. Indeed, it may even increase your difficulties in social situations because they become events to avoid rather than something you can, with the right skills, learn to manage successfully. If you could confidently break that cycle just by doing the things that make you anxious, however, you wouldn't be reading this book! Here we will describe the techniques that are most likely to help you reduce in a realistic way the extent to which you avoid challenging situations.

As you have worked through this book, we hope that you will have come to understand a great deal about your individual shyness or anxiety. The starting point for improving your confidence in social situations is to have a clear picture of what is most likely to make you feel shy or anxious and to work towards coping with the most challenging of those occasions in small steps. We can best show you this through case studies based on some of the people we have worked with.

> *Annie* was no longer invited to join her friends on outings where there would be more than three or four people. Although she enjoyed spending time with her friends in small groups, she found large groups, parties and formal occasions frightening. She would start to blush and stammer, thinking that everyone was looking at her and that they thought she was silly and uninteresting. After years of avoiding the

outings which scared her, Annie's best friend Natasha asked her to be chief bridesmaid. Annie agreed but became increasingly anxious at the prospect of being part of the wedding party and called Natasha one week later to pull out. Natasha was devastated and told Annie that it was time to seek professional help.

Annie became anxious in situations outside her home where more than three or four good friends were around. Being in familiar surroundings would help her remain calm to some extent, but she particularly dreaded being 'on show' to a large crowd as chief bridesmaid. Our experience has shown us that most people can cope with at least some social situations and that there are often particular features which identify the situations they struggle with most. These might be related to the number of people present, their role at that place and time or the nature of their surroundings. As you start to think about reducing your own avoidance, it is important to recognize what you can already do and what features of some situations make them especially challenging for you. Here are some examples to help you think about your unique difficulties:

- You may find situations at work more or less difficult than at home.
- There may be particular groups of people that you find especially challenging, perhaps doctors, teachers, managers, very confident friends or some relatives.
- Your shyness and anxiety may vary with the size of group you encounter: being lost in a crowd may seem easier than being the centre of attention. Alternatively, small groups may be less intimidating than large ones.

When Annie consulted her GP, he referred her to a psychologist and together they started to explore which situations were most likely to leave her feeling anxious and awkward. When they had listed these, Annie gave each one a score from 0 ('doesn't make me anxious at all') to 10 ('makes me extremely anxious'). Table 5.1 shows the list (sometimes called a 'fear hierarchy') they produced.

Table 5.1 Annie's fear list

Situation	Score
Meeting Natasha for lunch at a busy 'smart' restaurant I don't know well	3
Going shopping in a large complex with four or five friends	5
Going to a party at another friend's house	7
Joining in a karaoke evening for Natasha's hen night.	8
Being Natasha's chief bridesmaid	9

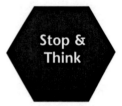

Can you construct your own fear hierarchy? Use the notes you made earlier to identify the situations most challenging for you, score them from 0 to 10 and put them in order.

Working with the psychologist, Annie decided that, although she found them uncomfortable, she could manage situations which scored less than 4 out of 10. She practised some relaxation techniques similar to those we describe later, and found that when she tried the first item on her list, meeting Natasha for lunch, she actually only became anxious enough to score 2 out of 10. This improved her confidence so that she was able to try the next challenge, shopping with a larger group of friends.

The first time Annie tried this, she felt very shy in a particularly smart shop and couldn't quite bring herself to try on a dress she really liked. Overall, she marked the experience as 6 out of 10 that time. After practising some other techniques similar to those in this book with the psychologist and at home, she tried again and found herself more confident, scoring 4 out of 10. With another two shopping trips, Annie reduced her score for this type of experience to 2 out of 10 and was ready to try the next step.

Fortunately, Annie's friends had several parties planned in the months before Natasha's wedding and Annie was able to practise the techniques she had learnt. At the first party, she stayed for just under an hour, chatted to the friends she knew best and went home feeling slightly ashamed that she had left early but having enjoyed some of the time she had been there. She built up her time and confidence gradually so that by the time of Natasha's karaoke party she was able to join in a duet of her favourite song and enjoy most of the night, with a score that reached a maximum of 4 out of 10. This gave her a useful boost for the wedding and she enjoyed being chief bridesmaid, scoring a maximum of 3 out of 10.

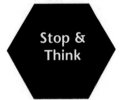

Stop & Think

What smaller challenges could you use to start building your confidence? What help do you need to tackle them? Could a friend come with you the first time, or could you perhaps use some of the relaxation techniques in the next chapter?

Annie's experience is unique but it does illustrate some things which are typical of many people we have worked with. As you work through your own fear hierarchy you may find that one or more of the steps you have planned become too great a challenge. If this happens, we would encourage you to persevere – not by trying to repeat the same thing, but by thinking about either asking for help and support to practise something that for now is too difficult on your own, or tackling a slightly less challenging task first. Here are some ways of doing this which might help:

- Did you attempt too big a step from your previous challenge? If this is the case you may be able to think of an intermediate step. For example, if you managed dinner with a few friends reasonably confidently but then found yourself overwhelmed with shyness at a party attended by 50 people, could you build up to that by going out with eight or nine friends and building up as your confidence improves?
- You may have rushed up your hierarchy too quickly. Don't be surprised if it takes several attempts at each stage to become confident. It is well worth spending time on each step to give yourself the chance to gain skills and confidence, making it more likely that you will successfully tackle the next challenge.
- Is there someone who could support you by coming with you and even reminding you of the skills in this book when you first attempt a new stage in your hierarchy?

As you work through your hierarchy, remember to reward yourself for each success and to treat what you may think of as failures as an opportunity to learn how to succeed next time. If you do find that this work becomes too difficult, you may find it useful to read Chapter 10 now.

6

Learning to relax

Learning relaxation skills is vital for treating social anxiety because it helps you to manage the bodily symptoms we described earlier. These skills will help you reduce and manage the physical sensations which play a large part in making shyness and anxiety feel so unpleasant. They will also help you to realize that you can cope with social situations. Learning how to control physical symptoms of anxiety is another skill that needs be practised frequently before you can expect lasting benefits. It can be difficult at first, especially if you try to apply relaxation skills during a challenging situation such as meeting new people or attending a dinner event. It is therefore important to begin your practice in settings where you feel comfortable.

This section presents a number of relaxation techniques that will help to reduce your anxiety, stress and tension. We first focus on relaxed, controlled ways of breathing before moving on to teaching you how to release physical tension and relax your body and mind. These are important skills that can help you feel calmer and more comfortable when you are with other people. Once you have learnt practical skills for reducing the bodily signs of anxiety, you will be in a much better frame of mind to focus your attention outwards and then tackle the unpleasant thoughts and behavioural elements thought to maintain your social anxiety. As with the techniques we described in the previous chapter, once you become skilled at relaxing, you can use the techniques here to counter the physical sensations you notice in difficult social situations.

Why learn to relax?

Although the physical experience of fear and anxiety is normal, it can cause high levels of discomfort if the reaction is misinterpreted or excessive. If your bodily reactions during a social situation – or, indeed, while worrying about an upcoming event – are extreme, the experience can be sufficiently frightening and distressing to give rise to two challenges: the unpleasant effects of anxiety coupled with a fear of experiencing these symptoms. These have the further effect of reinforcing one another. The anticipation of other people seeing your physical discomfort, nausea, sweating, breathing difficulties or tightening in the chest area, to name but a few, can then produce the stress that reinforces these bodily sensations. Table 6.1 shows an example of the many exaggerated interpretations of physical discomfort.

Table 6.1 Exaggerated interpretations of physical discomfort

Bodily changes	What is happening	Anxious thoughts
Shallow rapid breathing	Hyperventilation; you are using only the upper parts of the lungs and this results in the inhalation of too much oxygen	'I can't breathe', 'I am suffocating', 'Other people will be traumatized by watching me suffocating'
Muscle tightening in the chest area, headaches	Tension; muscular tension causes uncomfortable sensations such as headaches, tightness in chest area, pains, etc.	'This is a heart attack', 'I am having a stroke', 'I am drawing attention to myself'
Nausea and dizziness	When the oxygen level in your body rises (hyperventilation) the relative carbon dioxide level falls below normal. This imbalance causes unpleasant symptoms including nausea and light headedness	'I will collapse', 'I will faint', 'I will make a fool of myself'
Sweating, trembling, hot and flushed	The bodily temperature rises because of physical exertion brought on by hyperventilation and muscular tension	'I can't cope', 'Other people will see how weak and pathetic I really am'

There is a range of techniques that can help you to modify the bodily responses associated with social anxiety. We have found relaxed and controlled breathing and applied relaxation to be particularly effective ways of producing physical relief. These are widely recognized methods for coping with bodily sensations during anxiety attacks. They are designed to tackle hyperventilation (over-breathing) and muscle tension respectively. As we demonstrated in Table 6.1, the rapid shallow breathing and muscular tension are thought to maintain and reinforce many of the unpleasant sensations associated with your social anxiety. It therefore makes sense to deal with each of these in turn. You may already be familiar with breathing exercises and healthy ways of resting, especially if you practise yoga or meditation or have completed a course in relaxation skills. If this is the case, the techniques described below can be used to build on existing skills to enhance your repertoire for relaxation. You may find it helpful to record yourself or a trusted friend reading the instructions for each exercise so that you can play those instructions back to guide you as you practise.

Relaxed, controlled breathing

We tend to 'over-breathe' whenever we are tense, or when we are exercising. This is a mild form of hyperventilation, which increases blood circulation so that our muscles can be primed to react during activity. We notice that our heart rate increases, our breathing becomes more pronounced and our muscles may tense up slightly. Rapid breathing is not problematic in the short term. It is a perfectly healthy response to ensure we can sustain exercise, whether working out in the gym, running a marathon or speeding towards the office to make the morning meeting. It is also a normal response to stress and anxiety.

Continued rapid breathing can cause intense physical discomfort which can be quite frightening. Imagine that you are on your way to meet some old colleagues after work. Your breathing is getting heavier; you become hot and flushed. You may be thinking, 'What is happening to me?' and 'I am never going to feel normal around other people.' There are two things happening to your mind and body here: your initial worry of making a fool of yourself in front of your old colleagues has caused over-breathing which triggers off a range of physical sensations that can be quite uncomfortable; and these have led you to develop a second fear, 'I won't be able to control myself.' Although it is common to worry about losing control it is very unlikely that you will. It may feel as if the pain will never end and you may worry that you won't be able to restore healthy ways of breathing. This is a common response to continuous over-breathing. Being able to correct over-breathing is a very powerful way of reducing these unpleasant physical sensations.

You can easily learn to correct over-breathing by developing the habit of 'correct' breathing. Although breathing comes naturally and we all do it without even thinking, there is a tendency to lose our normal ways of breathing when we are afraid, such as fearing that others will judge us in a negative way. The breathing technique below will help you to develop the ability to control symptoms of over-breathing. You can apply the technique in almost any situation; during the lead-up to a social event, while popping to the loo in a restaurant or when seated at a dinner table with friends and family. The overall goal of this breathing technique is to learn a way to relax through breathing. This involves practising taking gentle, even breaths that fill your lungs completely and exhaling in a slow manner. You should start by practising this technique in a comfortable situation when you are not too stressed or anxious. Each exercise should last for about ten minutes and you should ideally practise twice a day if you can: once in the morning and once in the evening. Find a quiet place that is free from distractions and noise. This could be in your office, at home, in the garden or even at your local gym. When you first start practising, you may want to ensure you are alone as it is easy to lose focus when other people may distract you. You are also more likely to feel self-conscious if your partner or friend is watching when you practise relaxing and controlled breathing.

- Before you start, it is important that you feel comfortable and are able to relax. You can practise controlled breathing in a seated position with your hands relaxed on either side of your body, or with your back flat on the ground in a lying position. If you practise in a lying position, you might find it more comfortable to support your back by placing a pillow or cushion underneath your knees.

- Loosen any tight clothing and take off your shoes if you can.
- Let your shoulder blades sink down your back and lean slightly towards the back of the chair (or the ground if you're lying down) to support your back. Close your eyes.
- Start by taking a deep breath in through your nose and exhale slowly through your mouth. Continue to breathe in through your nose and out through your mouth about five more times.
- Try to make each inhalation and exhalation of the same duration. When you inhale, count slowly from 1 through to 4. Do the same when you exhale so that you are breathing evenly in a slow and focused manner. Notice how your breathing is slowing down.
- Feel the way your lungs gradually expand on every in breath. As you breathe out you are emptying your lungs. Your body feels relaxed. Continue to breathe slowly . . . in through your nose and out through your mouth.
- Place your right hand on your tummy and let it rest lightly on top of your navel. As you breathe in through your nose, feel the way your tummy rises. As you breathe out through your mouth, your hand is sinking further and further down towards the middle part of your body until your tummy feels completely flat.
- Your heartbeat is slowing down. Your arms and legs are relaxed. Continue to count slowly from 1 to 4 on each inhalation and then again for each exhalation.
- On each out breath, imagine that you are pushing the tension out of your lungs. Let it flow through your mouth and out into the wider world. You are getting rid of all the tension, stress and worry.
- Let go of all your bodily tension. Continue to breathe deeply five more times . . . in through your nose and out through your mouth. Feel the quietness and peacefulness around you.
- Slowly open your eyes. Continue to breathe gently and evenly in through your nose and out through your mouth. Softly move your legs and arms. Raise your arms upwards and stretch the whole of your body upwards if you are in a seated position. If you are lying down, flex your arms and legs downwards and gently move back up into a seated position.

You may find it a challenge to practise controlled breathing at first. It may feel as if you are not getting enough air, or that the pace of your breathing seems unnaturally slow. This is a normal reaction when you practise a new routine. If you find it difficult to read the instructions while carrying out the breathing routine (most of us do!), you may benefit from recording the instructions with lots of pauses and playing them back for the first few practices. As your skill improves and you learn to relax quickly, you will find it easier to switch to correct breathing whenever you feel anxious. You may want to progress to more distracting situations with your eyes open, such as getting the kids off to school, for example! This will improve your skills and help you to control your breathing before, during and after social situations. The technique is simple and can be used at any stage of a social experience. It is easy to apply and will help to reduce tension, anxiety and stress.

Releasing physical tension

Once you have learned the skill of relaxing your muscles, your mind and body will automatically feel calmer. It is almost imposs-ible for the mind to be tense when the body is relaxed. The ability to relax is not always something which comes easily; it is a skill that needs to be learnt gradually and practised regularly. As we have seen, anxiety is different for each of us. We may not have the same bodily symptoms; each of us has our own independent anxious thoughts and each of us behaves differently when under stress. It is therefore important that you find a relaxation technique that works for you. This is best done by regular practice before a social situation so that you get used to doing it and gain confidence in its benefits. The aim is to learn relaxation techniques in advance so that you are in a better position to manage your anxiety on the day of a social engagement. How quickly people can reduce the physical symptoms of anxiety varies from person to person. It will depend upon the severity of your anxiety, your ability to relax during stress and the nature of muscle tensions involved. Nevertheless, relaxation methods have a very good chance of success if you prac-tise them regularly and take them seriously.

Monitoring progress

Before you begin to practise relaxation skills, spend a minute or two on identifying the intensity of your stress and anxiety levels. This could be done by asking yourself: 'How tense/stressed/anxious do I feel right now?' Use a scale from 1 (low) to 10 (high) to rate the degree of tension/stress/anxiety.

Work through the first of the exercises provided below. Once you have finished the exercise, take a further measure of your anxiety. Compare the two sets of scores and see whether you feel less tense/anxious/stressed after completing the relaxation sequence, or whether there's no change. Repeat this procedure for each of the exercises provided. You need to know whether the relaxation procedure works for you, though there may be some minor variation from day to day.

Progressive muscular relaxation

The first exercise will help you to make a distinction between tensed and relaxed muscles. This will help you to identify when you are tense so that you can learn to relax your muscles. Muscular tension can occur automatically as a reaction to uncomfortable thoughts and worry. We are not always conscious of physical tension and it is therefore not uncommon for people to experience prolonged periods of muscular strain. This exercise will increase your awareness of bodily tension and can therefore act as a cue for when it may be beneficial to apply relaxation techniques to help let go of muscular strain. The sequence is quite simple and takes you through all parts of your body. This exercise is best done in a lying position, but if this is difficult sitting in a chair can work equally well. Once you are confident with the technique, you should practise it when sitting or standing as these are the positions you will mostly be in while attending social engagements. You can use the controlled breathing techniques in the previous exercise to enhance relaxation and calmness. Remember to make a note of how anxious/stressed you are before starting the exercise.

The basic movements which you can use for each part of your body are as follows: tense the muscles as much as you can and concentrate on feeling the strain within your body; hold the tension for about five seconds and then release your muscles; relax the muscle for 15 seconds and note the difference between the tense and relaxed state of your muscle. Use this basic technique on each of the muscle groups in turn. Remember to breathe gently and evenly throughout the exercise.

- *Hands* Clench your left hand and make a tight fist. Then relax your left hand – let it sink towards the ground. Do the same with your right hand.
- *Arms* Tense your whole arm. Imagine that you are holding a set of weights in your hand. Bring the bottom half of your arm upwards as this will make it easier to flex your arm. Relax for 15 seconds. Repeat the process for your other arm.
- *Face* Tense your eyebrows by frowning, then your forehead, then your jaws. Relax for 15 seconds and repeat.
- *Neck and shoulders* Let your chin drop down towards your chest. Squeeze your shoulders up towards your neck as hard as you can. Hold for 15 seconds and then relax. Repeat the process once more. As your shoulders release, feel your shoulder blades slide gently down your back towards your waist.
- *Abdomen* Tighten the muscles in your stomach by pulling them in and up. Relax for 15 seconds. Repeat the tensing and relax again.
- *Thighs* Relax your upper body. Tighten your thigh muscles by squeezing your buttocks and thighs together. Relax for 15 seconds before you repeat the process.
- *Legs* Bend your feet downwards so that your toes are pointing towards the floor. There should be a tightening sensation in the back of your leg muscles. Relax for 15 seconds. Then bend your feet the other way so that your toes are pointing upwards. You should feel a slight tension in the front part of your legs. Relax.
- *The whole of your body* Tense all of the above body parts all at once. You should feel a tension in your hands, face area, neck and shoulders, abdomen, thighs and legs. Relax for 15 seconds and then repeat this process once more.

Take care to not over-tense muscles as this can cause discomfort or even injury to your body. Remember to breathe slowly and regularly between each part of the exercise. When you have finished the sequence, spend a minute or two on thinking about something pleasant – for example, a relaxing walk along the seafront or eating a piece of your favourite chocolate cake. This can allow for a gentle transition back into your normal environment. Before you stand up straight, gently stretch and move your arms and legs and avoid sudden or jerky movements. When you are ready, take your time standing up. If you still feel tense at the end of the exercise try and go through the sequence once more. Remember, it takes time and practice to learn how to relax. Give yourself a chance and do not expect to master this straight away.

Once you have mastered this muscle-relaxing exercise, you can shorten it by missing out the tensing stage. You can go through the routine systematically by focusing on each of the muscle groups for 15–20 seconds at a time. You can adapt the exercise so that you can apply the relaxation procedure while at work, at home, during train journeys or anywhere else you can think of. Learning to relax in a range of different environments is important because this is what you need for coping in the real world. You can use relaxation skills at any point during the lead-up to an upcoming social event as well as on the day of social activities.

Deep relaxation

For this exercise, you will need to imagine a soothing, restful situation to use during the sequence. The mental image will help you relax even more effectively. This exercise is a form of distraction and can help people learn to calm themselves down. You may need to practise the sequence a number of times. This will help you to use a mental image to relax yourself while, for example, performing on a stage, hosting a dinner party or going on a date. Before you start the exercise, remember to note your anxiety/tension level and compare it with the level at the end. Here are some suggestions to help you get started:

- A particular place you have visited that you associate with peacefulness and calmness. This might be a deserted beach, your holiday home, your garden, the views from the top of a mountain, watching the rain drum against your window, the scenery during a visit to the countryside or any place you associate with peace and calm.

- A poem, lyric of a song, a word or a catch-phrase that brings positive images to your mind.
- A pleasant object, person, movie or picture that you particularly like.

When you have decided what mental image you will use, follow the instructions below. Again, it may be useful to record these, including lots of pauses, and to play the recording back to guide your first few practice sessions.

- Sit in a comfortable position with your eyes closed.
- Start by focusing on your breathing – listen to the sounds of your breaths.
- When you inhale, fill the lungs completely before you exhale by slowly letting go of the air. Slow the breathing down.
- As you continue to breathe, focus on your mental image: the things that you can see, hear and smell. Simply let go of all tension and allow your mind and body to relax.
- Feel your body growing heavier and heavier. Stay with the image and continue to breathe naturally and steadily. Keep the exercise going for 15–20 minutes.

When you have finished, open your eyes and sit in the same position for a minute or two. Slowly move your limbs and prepare yourself to stand up.

Relaxing in other situations

As we have seen, you can reduce self-consciousness by learning to redirect your attention away from your inner experience. When we are scared of a situation, our mind tends to attach unhelpful meanings to aspects of ourselves ('I can't cope', 'I am going to make a fool of myself', 'Other people think I am weird'), to the world around us ('Social events are dangerous and painful') and to other people ('People are judgemental, they are so much better than me').

Being able to pay less attention to our inward thoughts, emotions and physical sensations gives us more control over these anxious thoughts, and means that we have more capacity to react to what other people are saying and doing. Eventually this skill will make it easier for you to be more comfortable in social situations.

Learning how to relax is another important skill that can help reduce the bodily symptoms of social anxiety. As we have seen, controlled breathing and relaxation may need to be practised several times before you can expect to discover the effectiveness of their use. They are an important part of managing your social anxiety that can help reduce physical distress. For some people, the anticipation of physical symptoms can be more disturbing than the actual prospect of being with other people. In other words, they fear the upsetting experience of the fear! When you become skilled at relaxation techniques, you can be more confident in your ability to control those unpleasant sensations of anxiety in challenging situations. With practice, this will help to reduce the anxiety you feel in anticipation of symptoms such as blushing, stammering or feeling the need to break eye contact, because you can counter that anxiety by reminding yourself of the new tried and tested skills you have for controlling physical anxiety.

We now turn our attention to the role played by what you think in provoking and maintaining shyness or anxiety. The next chapters explain how thoughts may make a significant contribution to your difficulties and how to overcome this.

7

How does thinking drive my social anxiety?

The previous chapters have looked at what shyness is and asked you to think about your own experience of shyness and social anxiety in detail. We have also introduced the techniques which focus on what you can *do* to help improve your confidence and feel less anxious. This chapter explores the way in which what you think about yourself and social situations which you find difficult may be contributing to your anxiety. Once you've worked through this chapter, you will have more detailed information to help you to start identifying the ways you think that make you most anxious. Before we start, you might need to remind yourself of the links between thought and feelings we described earlier:

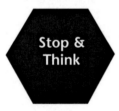

Remember from Chapter 4 that the way in which we think about an event can determine what we feel about it. For example, if you thought that a loud knock on the door was an unfriendly neighbour coming to complain, you'd probably be fairly anxious. On the other hand if you thought it was the postman delivering a parcel you wanted urgently, you might feel excited. Two different thoughts about the same event mean you feel very differently. Have another look at Figure 4.2 if you need to.

Two examples of social anxiety

Our experience and a large amount of published research have shown that what you think may be a major factor in your shyness or social anxiety. There are probably very good reasons why you think that way, and the earlier part of this book has described many of those. Thoughts which make you shy or anxious, however, are often unhelpful. Identifying and working with these thoughts is an effective way of coping with shyness. Before we explain this, we would like to introduce you to two case studies based on people we have worked with which we will use in this chapter to explain how thinking often drives social anxiety.

> *George* is a well-regarded software engineer who, as he put it, 'instinctively' turned down an offer of promotion to supervisor because the new role would involve managing people and contributing to departmental meetings. He said that when he had to consult with colleagues, he would think that they regarded him as 'a young upstart' who should do what his older colleagues told him and didn't have good ideas. This was in spite of glowing evaluations from George's manager and several successful solo projects. In situations like this, George would find himself anxious, stammering and critical of himself.

> *Mary* found herself increasingly dreading the annual family holiday. Sitting on a beach with her family was lovely. Having to deal with airline and hotel staff and other holidaymakers left her blushing, self-conscious, anxious and determined to send the family without her next time! When Mary needed to talk to strangers she would think that she appeared stupid and uninteresting to them – certainly not worth having a conversation with.

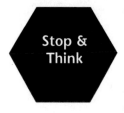

Stop & Think

Take a moment to see if you can identify the thoughts George and Mary had that helped to drive their social anxiety. Are they similar to some of the ways you think? If not, can you identify the way you think that might be contributing to your anxiety? Note these down; you'll find this useful information to work with later.

Mary thought that when she met people who did not know her well, they would regard her as stupid and uninteresting. George thought that his colleagues, who were generally about seven or eight years older, thought he was useless at his job. You will realize from your reading so far that these are thoughts and do not necessarily reflect the truth. As you also know, however, automatic thoughts such as these have a powerful effect on how we feel.

We will explore how Mary and George came to think this way and the impact of their thoughts later. Although their anxiety was triggered in very different situations, both came to think in ways which we find often maintain or reinforce feelings of anxiety or awkwardness in social situations. It is most frequently the result of a combination of wanting people to think well of us and thinking that we don't have the skills or confidence to make this happen. Somehow, people will just look through us, or worse. In general, this often works as we've illustrated in Figure 7.1.

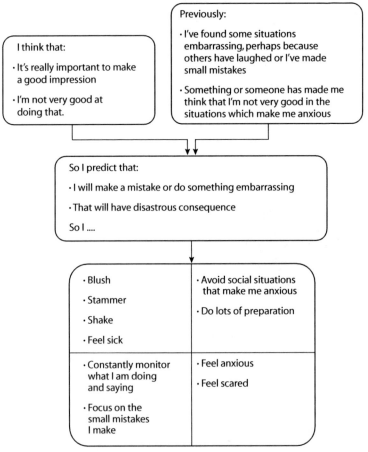

Figure 7.1 Thinking and social anxiety

Thinking and social anxiety

Figure 7.1 shows that people who are anxious in social situations feel that way because it is really important to them to make a good impression. They focus more on this need than almost anything else. For some, including Mary, it's particularly important that people like them. Others, like George, think that they need to appear good at what they do. Remember that wanting to make a good impression is generally a good thing. The people who come to us asking for help with their shyness just go a little further than people who do not experience this form of anxiety. We find that this way of thinking often goes hand in hand with the view that you do not have the skills to handle the social situations that make you anxious. Remember the link between thoughts and feelings we described earlier? In any situation that makes you think this way, you have no choice but to be anxious! In the next chapter, we'll show you how to work with the way you think to reduce your anxiety. For now, the good news is that (whatever you might be thinking right now!) it is possible to change the way you think, and that will produce changes in the way you feel.

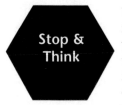

Stop & Think

When you look at Figure 7.1, can you identify similar ways of thinking which you notice yourself using in social situations? Try and remember the last time you felt shy. What were you thinking and how did that make you feel? Take a few moments to note down the thoughts you can remember. This will be useful in the next chapter.

When people first ask for psychological help with social anxiety, they have often had months or even years of 'practice' at feeling truly awful in the situations that scare them. Other people, places or events might have 'helped' reinforce this. For example, Mary told us that she moved every year or so throughout her school years. She was labelled 'stupid' by many pupils and some teachers every year because her education was so disrupted that she was always genuinely behind with her studies. By the time she was 13,

Mary had stopped trying to make friends because she found that many people laughed at her in school. Later, when she consulted a counsellor, Mary was able to see how these experiences made situations like holidays so difficult.

George, in contrast, had always been reasonably confident until he started work. When he was selected for accelerated training in his job, he was allocated to a department where his colleagues were older and initially made many jokes about the 'young upstart' joining them. George and his psychologist came to the conclusion that this was probably part of the reason he became anxious at work.

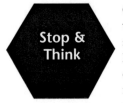

Can you think of previous experiences which might have contributed to your social anxiety? It's not always necessary to know why you've become anxious, so don't worry if you can't. The CBT techniques in this book are based on what you think and do now.

Understanding what we think

Hopefully, we have by now convinced you that what you think has a powerful effect on your emotions, physical reactions and even behaviour. We often find that people struggle to identify what they are thinking and therefore find it very difficult to work with the techniques we will describe in the next chapter. If you find yourself in this situation, it is unlikely that you are especially insensitive, unaware or stupid. It is a difficulty that many people have because we do not generally pay much attention to consciously noting each of our thoughts. Indeed, it is often useful to be able to think unconsciously and this often has good results: it is how we drive a car, ride a bicycle and talk to friends! You could picture our thoughts as an iceberg where we are only aware of the small portion above the surface – what we can consciously recognize. A much larger proportion of our thoughts are unconscious, and we may not immediately be aware of them.

Thoughts that we find difficult to bring into consciousness can have a significant impact on social anxiety and shyness. If you start to work with thoughts and find that they are difficult to challenge, it may be that spending some time exploring what these thoughts mean to you may help identify what you are thinking below the surface. Psychologists often use a technique called the 'downward arrow' to do this. Essentially, if you are struggling to see how a particular thought has such an impact on your emotions, use these steps:

1 Write the thought down. Simply having to put a thought into words or seeing it in writing can help clarify what it means to you.
2 Ask yourself, 'If that is true, what does it mean about me, the world I live in and the future?' Draw an arrow below your first thought and write this meaning beneath it.
3 Keep on doing this until you come to a way of expressing the thought that seems to summarize what drives your anxiety.

You will know when to stop for two reasons: (1) if you ask, 'If it is true what does it mean?' again, you will get the answer you already have; (2) the thought you have ended up with will seem very powerful to you and may make you anxious, sad or even angry. If that happens, take a break and do something relaxing before you come back to this book. Here is an example of Mary using the technique with her thought, 'People will think I am uninteresting and stupid.'

- 'People on holiday will think I am uninteresting and stupid.'
  - If this is true, what does it mean about me, the world I live in and the future?

- 'I am uninteresting and stupid.'
  - If this is true, what does it mean about me, the world I live in and the future?

- I will always be left out and isolated.
  - If this is true, what does it mean about me, the world I live in and the future?

- I am not worth getting to know.

Once Mary had realized why her thoughts had such an impact on how she felt, she was able to start working with them as we describe later. If you find that challenging unhelpful thoughts using those techniques is not as successful as you would like, it may be useful to review the thoughts you are working with using this downward arrow technique.

Why am I still anxious?

So far in this chapter, you will have identified some of the thinking that encourages you to be anxious in the social situations that you find difficult. We find that, almost always, there's a bit more to it: as people, our brains and the way we think are very focused on trying to keep us safe and comfortable. If there's a situation that makes us anxious, we will tend to think that we should avoid it. Look again at the bottom box in Figure 7.1. Those thoughts, feelings, physical reactions and behaviours do not feel safe or comfortable, and our thinking and actions will be very focused on keeping us safe. Later chapters will look at managing actions and physical reactions.

When we start to learn almost anything, as children or adults, we quickly discover that 'practice makes perfect', so we rehearse, practise and focus on monitoring what we do until we get it 'right'. Particularly when we are children, it's often the adults around us who point out small mistakes and show us the correct way to do things. As we get older, we learn to monitor what we do ourselves and often become our own instructor as we learn even more skills. There's nearly always someone else around who will comment on our performance as well and that's usually helpful in gaining skill and confidence.

Rehearsing and practising is generally helpful. We often find, however, that one of the ways in which anxious people understandably think in challenging situations causes them to take that just a bit too far. It then becomes another way of thinking that helps them remain anxious.

> If she was forced into a situation where she had to try and talk to people she didn't know, Mary would focus on her own facial expression and body language and on rehearsing her reply in an attempt to seem

intelligent and interesting. While this might seem a sensible way to focus attention on what she was doing, Mary discovered that she was constantly criticizing herself. This meant that she didn't have the capacity to focus on other people and frequently missed what they were saying. She would then feel that she really was stupid for not keeping up with the conversation and would resolve to focus even harder on her behaviour in future.

We often find that this sort of vicious cycle is remarkably effective in increasing anxiety. Another common vicious cycle centres on the way in which we think about the physical reactions which are so obvious to us in anxiety-provoking situations.

George became determined to stop stammering around his work colleagues and would practise for hours at home. As soon as he felt anxious at work, however, he would start to stammer. He noticed that he tended to think that this meant he must be very anxious. This would increase his anxiety and he would stammer even more.

We have drawn these two common vicious cycles of thoughts in Figure 7.2.

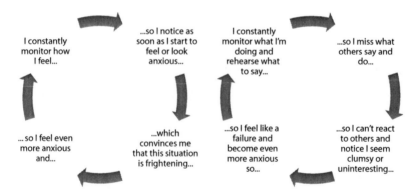

Figure 7.2 Vicious cycles of anxious thinking

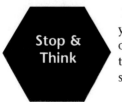

Stop &
Think

Finally for this chapter, try and draw out your unique cycles of anxiety. How much of your attention is focused on monitoring what you are doing? What does this stop you noticing?

It is well worth taking the time to work through this chapter and think about your individual way of thinking in anxious situations. Understanding how you think will help you select the techniques from the next chapter which are most likely to help you think differently. That in turn will help you to feel less anxious.

8

How thinking differently can help me manage my social anxiety

The previous chapter showed you how the ways in which you think may increase your feelings of anxiety in social situations. Now that you have a clearer understanding of your unique social anxiety, you can begin to select and learn the techniques most likely to work for you. As we described earlier, almost everyone who wants to become more confident in social situations will need to work on what they think and do and how their body reacts to anxiety or shyness. This chapter illustrates skills and techniques for working with what you think. We especially focus on how you might think about blushing or stammering, as these are often the symptoms which cause most distress for people who are shy or socially anxious.

Can I really change thoughts that make me shy or anxious?

It may seem daunting or even impossible to change the way in which you think, but don't be deterred. First of all, remember that what we are asking you to do is learn a new skill. Think back to learning to ride a bicycle or drive a car, or starting a new hobby. Most people need a lot of practice to become skilled at anything. Managing the way in which you think involves learning another new skill, and almost nobody will be perfect at it to start with. Second, you will find as you work through this chapter that the techniques we will share with you here are about spotting and challenging unhelpful ways of thinking. The aim is not to control what you think; rather, it is to identify and then work with unhelpful ways of thinking when they do happen so that you can change how you feel and reduce your anxiety and shyness.

The rest of this chapter explains the techniques most likely to help you manage thoughts and beliefs which increase or maintain anxiety or shyness. In summary, these are the basic steps to managing the thoughts which may drive social anxiety:

- Notice thoughts which make you feel shy or anxious.
- Check how accurate those thoughts are.
- If they are accurate, techniques that may help are those which focus on what you do.
- If these thoughts do not help you to feel confident in social situations, use the techniques in this chapter to challenge them and monitor the effect this has on your anxiety.

Most people we have worked with found that they needed to manage both what they do and how they think. You will probably find that you will need both types of technique as well.

Notice thoughts which make you feel shy or anxious

As you worked through the previous chapter, you will have gained a good understanding of the ways in which you tend to think which may contribute towards making you feel anxious in situations you find difficult. The starting point is to notice these thoughts and the context in which they occur, such as the places, people or events that trigger them. It's also important to identify the way these thoughts make you feel.

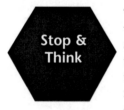

Take the time to identify the situations where you are most likely to become anxious, what you think then and how that makes you feel. You may find it useful to make your own version of the thought record used in the following examples and complete the first three columns using situations where you feel anxious over the next few days. Remember that thoughts may consist of words or they may be images in your mind.

George and Mary both found using thought records useful. Tables 8.1 and 8.2 show some examples of the first three columns of their early records.

Table 8.1 Thought records: Mary

	Example from Mary	
Situation	Thoughts or images	Mood
Having dinner with friends. Jane asked what holiday plans we had for next summer. Gordon (my husband) said he would like to go to the Caribbean and stay in a luxury hotel with different water sports.	If I tried to learn to water-ski or windsurf, I can picture me blushing in front of the instructor and falling off. I'd be no good at all. Hotels like that have lots of guests and staff around. I won't know what to say to them and I'll look stupid	Anxious (90/100) Ashamed (80/100)

Table 8.2 Thought records: George

	Example from George	
Situation	Thoughts or images	Mood
In a team meeting at work trying to describe how I'd solved a problem last week.	I can 'see' myself stammering and looking like an idiot. Everyone thinks I took too long to solve this problem	Anxious (95/100) Angry (70/100) Self conscious (80/100)

Mary was thinking about something that hadn't happened yet while George recorded what he thought and felt about a difficult situation at work. They both managed to identify the way they thought and linked that to the way they felt about challenging situations. Mary was particularly anxious about blushing while George worried about stammering.

Check how accurate your thoughts are

When we concentrate on trying to get something right or appearing skilled and confident, we tend not to pay very much attention to what we are thinking. That means that thoughts like 'I'll look stupid' or 'I can't explain myself properly' go unnoticed and make us feel anxious, ashamed or even angry. When trying to treat social anxiety, it's important to notice these thoughts and check how accurate they are. Look for the evidence which supports or contradicts the way you have been thinking.

If you find this difficult, you may find it helpful to remember the ways of thinking we described in Chapter 7, which often increase anxiety in social situations:

- 'It's really important to make a good impression.'
- 'I'm not very good at doing that.'

We also find that it's often helpful to know about common errors in the way that we think:

1 *All-or-nothing thinking*: a tendency to think in absolute or extreme terms about a situation, mostly in a negative way. For example: 'Everybody's looking at me' or 'I always stammer at work.'

2 *Negative focus*: focusing on negative or upsetting experiences or thoughts while ignoring other aspects that paint a different picture of the situation. One example is: 'I'm blushing,' when people are enjoying the funny story you're telling and may not even notice.

3 *Jumping to conclusions or mind reading*: a tendency to assume that the worst will happen in spite of a lack of evidence to support it. For example: 'I know I'll stammer all through dinner with my husband's colleagues even though last time I only stammered a little and no one seemed to notice.'

4 *Catastrophizing*: negative characteristics of a person or situation are exaggerated, however unlikely they are. For example: 'The fact that my boss looked at his watch while I was speaking meant he thought my ideas were rubbish,' when actually he had to watch the time because he had a flight to catch.

5 *Living by fixed rules*: thoughts are somehow distorted which tend to 'fix' people rigidly in a situation, making it seem that they are governed by quite extreme or inflexible rules. For example: 'I should be able to cope with this. I shouldn't have any unpleasant feelings. It must be because I haven't practised enough. I have

to give up my job.' Readers may be amused by the slight irreverence of a famous therapist called Albert Ellis, who termed this tendency 'musterbation'.

6 *Personalization or attribution*: exaggerating causation when the facts do not necessarily support this. For example: 'I started to explain something and everyone looked away – I must have been boring,' when someone's mobile phone had rung and distracted everyone.

(Based on David Burns, *Feeling Good: The new mood therapy*, New York, Plume, 1999)

These errors are the most common ways in which thoughts can become unhelpful and make us feel anxious.

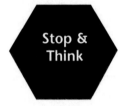

Stop & Think

Take a few moments now to look at your own thought records and see if you can spot any of these errors in your own thinking. If you haven't had the chance to start your own records yet, try working with the examples from Mary and George.

Mary and George were able to identify some errors in the thoughts they identified: see Tables 8.3 and 8.4.

Both George and Mary initially needed help to spot the errors in their thoughts, so don't be surprised if you find this difficult. It is often more straightforward to challenge unhelpful thoughts by looking at the evidence for and against them. It is important to pay just as much attention to the evidence for unhelpful thoughts as the evidence against them: otherwise you'll end up trying to think in unrealistically positive ways and that will not help. We will show you more on looking for evidence shortly, but first Tables 8.5 and 8.6 show what Mary and George came up with for one of each of their unhelpful thoughts:

In Tables 8.5 and 8.6, both Mary and George were able to notice the way that other people behaved. That can often be a very useful starting point. Other types of evidence that might be useful include:

- Formal appraisals at work
- Feedback from friends and family, for example being invited to join in social activities

Table 8.3 Errors in thinking: Mary

Example from Mary			
Situation	Thoughts or images	Mood	Possible errors
Having dinner with friends. Jane asked what holiday plans we had for next summer. Gordon (my husband) said he would like to go to the Caribbean and stay in a luxury hotel with different water sports.	If I tried to learn to water-ski or windsurf, I can picture me blushing in front of the instructor and falling off. I'd be no good at all.	Anxious (90/100) Ashamed (80/100)	Negative focus Catastrophizing
	Hotels like that have lots of guests and staff around. I won't know what to say to them and I'll look stupid.		Catastrophizing

Table 8.4 Errors in thinking: George

Example from George			
Situation	Thoughts or images	Mood	Possible errors
In a team meeting at work trying to describe how I'd solved a problem last week.	I can 'see' myself stammering and looking like an idiot.	Anxious (95/100) Angry (70/100)	Negative focus Personalization
	Everyone thinks I took too long to solve this problem.	Self-conscious (80/100)	Catastrophizing

- Other people's reactions when you are talking
- Seeing yourself in video and photographs

Notice that this type of evidence needs you to pay attention to other people's reactions rather than inwardly focus on your thoughts and feelings. This is another reason why it is often important to work on reducing self-consciousness if you are shy: allowing feelings of

Table 8.5 Challenging unhelpful thoughts: Mary

		Example from Mary		
Situation	Thoughts or images	Mood	Possible errors	Evidence
Having dinner with friends. Jane asked what holiday plans we had for next summer. Gordon (my husband) said he would like to go to the Caribbean and stay in a luxury hotel with different water sports.	If I tried to learn to water-ski or windsurf, I can picture me blushing in front of the instructor and falling off. I'd be no good at all.	Anxious (90/100) Ashamed (80/100)	Mental filter Catastrophizing	**For:** Last holiday I felt stupid and blushed when the couple next to us on the flight tried to talk to us. **Against:** They asked us to go sailing with them later that week and we had a good time. I even got to steer the boat back into harbour.

self-consciousness to keep your attention focused on yourself means that you will not see the clues that others may actually think well of you.

Most people find it much easier to find the evidence that supports unhelpful thoughts than evidence that might contradict that way of thinking. These questions may help you identify evidence which doesn't support thoughts that make you feel anxious:

- Can you think of any experiences which show that thought isn't completely correct at all times? (This question helped Mary to remember the enjoyable day sailing with people she met on holiday.)
- If a good friend or loved one thought this way, what would I say to him or her?

Table 8.6 Challenging unhelpful thoughts: George

		Example from George		
Situation	Thoughts or images	Mood	Possible errors	Evidence
In a team meeting at work trying to describe how I'd solved a problem last week.	I can 'see' myself stammering and looking like an idiot.	Anxious (95/100)	Mental filter Personalization	**For:** I did stammer **Against:** No one commented on my stammer or looked annoyed. Alan my manager said he'd like me to write up my solution to include it in the department newsletter.

- What did other people actually say about how I appeared in the situation that worried me? (This question helped George notice the positive responses from his manager and colleagues.)
- If I made a mistake or appeared awkward, stammering or blushing, did that really matter? Did everyone really notice? If they did notice, were they sympathetic or critical? (If you've ever watched somebody who gets anxious speaking in public, for example, did you feel sympathetic or annoyed?)

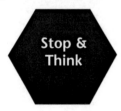
**Stop &
Think**

Do you notice how almost all these sources of evidence are based on what other people think? Often when people become anxious or shy in social situations, they focus so intently on what's going on in their thoughts and physical reactions that they filter out reactions from others around them which could well be positive. In his meeting at work, for example, George was so worried that he might be blushing that he didn't notice that most of his colleagues were nodding and taking notes – evidence that they probably thought his solution was a good one. Take a few moments to think about who you could ask for objective feedback on how you appear in situations where you feel anxious, or what evidence you could gather about the unhelpful thoughts you have noted so far.

Working with the evidence for and against unhelpful thoughts

It's important not to rush gathering evidence to support or challenge the way in which you think. Once you have collected all the evidence you can, look through it as objectively as possible. It may help if you ask someone you trust to do this with you to start with. If you do this, explain that you need the person to be objective. He or she will want to support you and may worry about hurting your feelings if there is evidence to back up your upsetting thoughts. You may find it useful to work through Chapter 9 with whoever is helping you first. We often find it's particularly helpful to remind someone who wants to help you that you need to understand how accurate your thoughts are so that you can decide how to work with them. If they are accurate then the 'doing' techniques we described earlier are designed to help you work with what you do. If they have some errors, the techniques in this chapter will help you construct more realistic ways of thinking.

As you look at the evidence you have collected, ask yourself:

- Is there more evidence for or against that way of thinking?
- When you look at the evidence objectively, how accurate is that thought?
- Can you identify any errors in the way you are thinking?
- Is there another way to think about it?

Once you have taken the time to look at the evidence in detail, you will often see that the thought which makes you feel anxious, ashamed or unhappy isn't completely accurate.

About blushing and stammering

Blushing and stammering are reactions to feeling shy, embarrassed or anxious which we cannot completely control. They are part of the physical reaction to anxiety described earlier. What we do have a degree of control over is the way in which we think about blushing or stammering. In turn, that gives us some control over what we feel when this happens to us. If you can work with how you manage your reaction to blushing or stammering, you will improve your confidence and the result is often that you blush or stammer less frequently.

The most common response to blushing or stammering is to catastrophize: to think that these involuntary responses are a disaster socially. While it is understandable that you might think this way, it will increase your feelings of anxiety and shame and it is probable that you will overestimate the extent to which other people think badly of you or even notice.

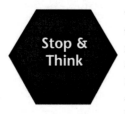 What do you imagine other people think when you find yourself blushing or stammering? Often, people who are socially anxious think that everyone in the room notices and thinks negatively about them. Actually, it may be that very few people notice and those who do are likely to be sympathetic. Remember that they are likely to be shy or awkward in some situations as well. If you are worried about how you appear to others, it may be useful to ask a few trusted friends what they think if they notice that someone is blushing or stammering.

You will see how Mary and George constructed alternative ways of thinking about stammering or blushing. One additional technique that we sometimes find helpful is to 'name' what is happening in order to reduce the extent to which you are focusing on your internal reactions. You might, for example, say, 'Oops, there I go stuttering again as I get excited about . . .' Most people will respond sympathetically and you may find this improves your confidence.

Table 8.7 Alternative ways of thinking: Mary

		Example from Mary			
Situation	Thoughts or images	Mood then	Evidence	Alternative thought	Mood now
Having dinner with friends. Jane asked what holiday plans we had for next summer. Gordon (my husband) said he would like to go to the Caribbean and stay in a luxury hotel with different water sports.	If I tried to learn to water-ski or windsurf, I can picture me blushing in front of the instructor and falling off. I'd be no good at all.	Anxious (90/100) Ashamed (80/100)	**For:** Last holiday I felt stupid and blushed when the couple next to us on the flight tried to talk to us. **Against:** They asked us to go sailing with them later that week and we had a good time. I even got to steer the boat back into harbour.	I can't control my blushing but I can try and change my reaction to it. No one mentioned it on our last holiday and they seemed sympathetic and enjoyed my company.	Anxious (30/100) Excited (60/100)

Table 8.8 Alternative ways of thinking: George

		Example from George			
Situation	Thoughts or images	Mood then	Evidence	Alternative thought	Mood now
In a team meeting at work trying to describe how I'd solved a problem last week.	I can 'see' myself stammering and looking like an idiot.	Anxious (95/100) Calm (70/100)	**For:** Geoff called me 'young upstart' yesterday **Against:** Alan my manager doesn't look annoyed and after the meeting said he'd like me to write up my solution to include it in the department newsletter.	Nobody really seemed to pay much attention to my stammer and they all took an interest in my solution. No one interrupted me and Alan obviously thought I'd done well.	Anxious (40/100) Calm (70/100)

Construct alternative ways of thinking

The final step in working with unhelpful thoughts is to practise alternative ways of thinking about the situations which triggered those thoughts. Again this takes practice and can seem challenging at first, and you may want to ask someone you trust to help. The most important thing to remember is that we're not asking you to come up with 'empty' positive ways of thinking. Any alternative must be based on the evidence you collected when challenging this thought – it has to be realistic. Then notice how the alternative way of thinking makes you feel.

See Tables 8.7 and 8.8 for some examples from Mary and George.

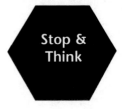

Notice that the alternative ways of thinking didn't completely take away the anxiety that Mary and George felt. More realistic thinking did reduce their anxiety, however, and helped Mary to realize that she could look forward to meeting new people on holiday. George was able to notice signs that his colleagues and manager thought he was good at his job.

Mary struggled to come up with an alternative way of thinking, and it was only when her psychologist asked about positive experiences on her last holiday that she was able to complete the example above. You may find it helpful to think about situations where you do feel confident and how you think then. One of the clients we have worked with, for example, became very anxious on business trips abroad because he found it embarrassing to try and use even short phrases in other languages. He thought his accent was bad and found meeting foreign customers very difficult as he became embarrassed at what he thought of as slow and laboured attempts at communication. His children, however, would always ask him to read them a particular set of stories because he was really good at the sounds and animal voices! When he was able to start thinking about imitating foreign accents in the same way as reading those stories and realized that his customers didn't expect him to be fluent, but appreciated small attempts at greetings in their language, he became more relaxed. As often happens, the social situations he found particularly awkward were limited to a particular context (meeting foreign customers) and he had skill in other situations (telling stories to his children) which helped his anxiety.

George realized that when he paid attention to the way his colleagues reacted, rather than how he felt, he was able to see that they appreciated his skills at work. As we described earlier, it is often helpful to focus 'outside' ourselves rather than 'inside' in such situations. This allows us to gather more objective evidence about how we appear to others.

When trying to construct alternative ways of thinking in difficult situations, start by taking an objective look at all the evidence you have gathered. Does it really prove that the thoughts you are working with are completely true all the time? If those thoughts are accurate, you may want to put this work to one side and either review Chapters 5 and 6 or move on to Chapter 10. If the evidence shows that they're not absolutely correct all the time, then constructing an alternative thought based on all the evidence and practising that way of thinking is very likely to reduce your anxiety. You may find it helpful to review Chapter 7 if you find it difficult to design alternative ways of thinking. The following questions and list of examples may also help.

- Did I fall into the trap of using any of the common errors in thinking?
- What would somebody who was more confident in that situation be thinking?
- Was I so focused on the fact that I felt anxious, awkward or stupid that I didn't notice that at least some people reacted positively to me or what I was saying?
- If I received formal or informal feedback from other people, what did they think was good about what I did?
- If I do feel nervous, awkward or even physically sick, does it really last for ever?
- When I look back in five years' time, how important will that situation be?

Table 8.9 shows examples of thoughts that clients we have worked with identified as unhelpful and the alternatives they constructed.

Table 8.9 Unhelpful thoughts and alternative thoughts based on evidence

Automatic or unhelpful thought	Alternative thought based on evidence
'I'm blushing or stammering and everyone thinks I'm incompetent.'	'Has everyone really noticed? Are they disdainful or sympathetic? I can't control these automatic reactions but I can focus on something else for a while and see if that helps me to calm down.'
'I feel stupid and awkward.'	'These feelings are uncomfortable but they won't last long and if I focus on what other people around me are saying or doing I'll feel less awkward'.
'Everyone's looking at me.'	'There are probably at least a few people who are planning what to cook for dinner or what to get in the shops. If they are looking at me it's because I'm saying something interesting'.
'I'll make a mistake.'	'Nobody expects me to be completely perfect all the time. If I make a small mistake I can correct it and carry on. Most people won't even notice.'
'I can't cope.'	'Even though I blushed and stammered last time, it was over quite quickly and nothing truly awful happened.'
'Everyone else always seems to be confident doing this.'	'So many people are anxious or shy in situations which involve interacting with others that I am not the only one who feels anxious or shy doing this. Most people will be sympathetic if they notice I look awkward and I have practised how to cope.'
'If I am not perfect, something terrible will happen.'	'Exactly what might happen? Even if I am not perfect, how many people will really notice and will it matter in five years' time?'

Realistic alternative ways of thinking can have a significant impact on the way we feel about situations and people we find difficult. It often takes practice both to construct the alternative thoughts and to use them in challenging situations. Remember that you may have had years of practice in unhelpful ways of thinking and it will take time to recognize and change those thoughts.

Putting it into practice

As we have said before, many people we have worked with have tried many solutions to their shyness before they decided to seek help from a counsellor or psychological therapist. They have often put a lot of time and energy into solutions which have not been successful and will, understandably, have become disheartened. Here is another example based on several people we have worked with.

> Maureen said that she had been shy for as long as she could remember. She found it difficult to be in any situation where she had to talk to another person, especially if she didn't know that person well. She would blush, think that she appeared stupid and feel very anxious about taking part in conversations. She had read several books on improving social skills and put a lot of effort into putting the suggestions in those books into practice.
>
> When Maureen first met with a psychologist, he noticed that she appeared very anxious talking to him. She often asked him to repeat questions and seemed to alternate her gaze fixedly between him and the wall behind him. When the psychologist mentioned this to Maureen, she said that she was concentrating on putting the social skills she had learnt into practice. Maureen described how she would look at the person she was talking to while she mentally counted to seven, then look away while she counted three, and then look back again. She was trying to maintain eye contact without being intimidating, something she had read in a book. Unfortunately, using so much of her attention on maintaining eye contact and thinking about how she appeared meant that Maureen often appeared uninterested in other people, especially as she frequently didn't hear what they said and therefore found it difficult to take part in interesting conversations.
>
> Working with her psychologist, Maureen was able to challenge her unhelpful thoughts and reduce her self-consciousness. With practice,

she found that she became less anxious and naturally looked at people she was talking with in an engaging way, without consciously having to time eye contact.

Maureen's story and those of many people we have worked with have shown us how important it is to work with what you think and what you do. They also illustrate how solutions which do not work as we would like often provide information which helps find a more useful way to cope with shyness.

Summary

There's a lot of information in this chapter and you may need to come back to it more than once. Essentially, we have shown you that there are ways in which you can change how you feel by working with what you think. The basic steps are:

1 Identify the situations which you find difficult and make a note of what you think then and how that makes you feel.
2 Take an objective look at those thoughts. Can you see any thinking errors? What is the evidence?
3 If the thinking is accurate (for example, you were stammering quite a lot) use the techniques in Chapters 5 and 6 to change what you do.
4 If the thinking isn't completely accurate, how else could you think about the evidence you have collected? Practise that new way of thinking and notice how it makes you feel.

9

How to help a friend or a relative with social anxiety

Many clients we treat for social anxiety describe how difficult it can be for others to understand how to help them. As we have seen in this book, if a close friend or family member has social anxiety there are many challenges that he or she will face. Having a supportive family and network of friends can make it easier to cope with and overcome social anxiety. For a start, support and understanding can help to reduce your fears, embarrassment and feelings of shame. Learning to cope successfully with shyness requires hard work from you and a great deal of patience from your family and friends.

It is not always easy for family members or friends to know exactly what they can do to help someone overcome difficulties with social anxiety. That said, the first thing they can do to help is to take the anxious person and his or her shyness seriously, be supportive and help reduce feelings of vulnerability and fear. However, they must not fully collude with avoidance or no progress will be made. This chapter will show friends and relatives how to support someone who becomes anxious in social situations, using the techniques described in this book. If you have worked through this book and want to ask a friend or a relative to help you put the techniques we described into practice, you could start by lending your friend this book and suggesting that he or she reads this chapter first. If you are trying to support someone who has asked you for help in reducing his or her social anxiety, this chapter is a good starting point.

If a friend or a relative has asked you to help with an issue like social anxiety, you may feel overwhelmed or think that you have no idea what to do. This chapter is written specifically for you, to give some specific ways of providing support, but there is a lot of information in the earlier part of the book that may be useful too. You may want to read some of those chapters to help you understand your friend or relative's difficulties. Perhaps you could ask which chapters have been most useful and suggest that your friend teaches you about his or her unique social anxiety. If you do feel overwhelmed, remember that social anxiety is a very treatable psychological difficulty, but if you are not a qualified therapist or psychologist it would be unreasonable to expect you to deliver 'therapy'. You may need to encourage your friend or relative to seek professional help, and the next chapter has more information on when to do that. Remember, however, that social anxiety often makes it difficult to ask for help – it is doing the very thing that the person is scared of, such as making social contact about something that may feel shameful or embarrassing. Someone who has asked you for help has recognized that he or she is unable to overcome this difficulty alone. That is a good starting point.

A brief introduction to social anxiety

There are a variety of ways to support someone with social anxiety. The most effective way to help a person manage his or her fear of social situations will of course depend upon the particular situations that person finds challenging. No two people are exactly the same and it is therefore important to understand that not everyone with social anxiety will experience the exact same difficulties.

> *Tina*, for example, has never plucked up the courage to go on a date because she is convinced that other people think she is boring, unattractive and un-cool. She does not want to be single but the fear of exposing herself to negative evaluations of her appearance is too frightening for Tina to bear.

> *Linda*, on the other hand, calls in sick once a month to avoid the monthly team meetings at her work. She is convinced that her colleagues will laugh at her ideas, thinking that they are stupid and ridiculous.

> *Felix* avoids making eye contact with his professor during lectures because he is petrified of being called on, even when he knows the answers. He is afraid that his whole class will see how anxious he is and notice his blushing and that he will become monosyllabic, and they will therefore think of him as 'weak' and 'pathetic'.

Starting to support someone with social anxiety

As we can clearly see, the symptoms and causes of social anxiety vary greatly between people, though a strong fear of negative outcomes connects them together. It is therefore important that you seek to understand the unique nature of your friend or relative's difficulties. When you can sit calmly together, these questions may help you understand:

- What situations does your friend fear?
- What does your friend fear could happen to him or her?
- What does he or she think makes these situations especially difficult?
- What has your friend tried to do to solve this difficulty?
- What has helped? Has anything made him or her more anxious?

Don't be afraid to ask your friend how he or she would like you to give support.

We may sometimes assume that we know what our partner, close friend or family member needs, and this can lead to misunderstandings, even if our actions are carried out with the best of intentions. One person, for example, may prefer to be accompanied during an anxiety-provoking situation, whereas someone else will prefer to face the challenge alone, or just avoid it altogether. What essentially is preferred, desired or needed by one individual may not necessarily be the same for another. It is therefore helpful that you and the person with social anxiety work together to establish how much or how little he or she would want you to be involved in the exposure and treatment.

There is a great deal of information in books and online about social anxiety. We hope this book helps to consolidate and synthesize much of what is known, and is of practical value. Take the time to learn as much as you can in order to better understand the condition. This can be a helpful way of letting someone know that you are interested in his or her shyness and that you want to help. Simply acknowledging that you know your partner, friend, child or relative experiences social anxiety can be validating and supportive. As we have already stated, this can help remove or relieve feelings of shame or embarrassment with at least one other person, which can be therapeutic. When the condition has been evident for quite a long time before it is diagnosed, both the person and his or her friends may come to see this as 'just a negative personality trait'. Take a look at the following example:

When Mohammed was at school, he used to spend the majority of his lunch breaks in the library. He was terrified of meeting new pupils and 'having' to fit in a group, fearing that they would judge him in a negative way. At home, he would make excuses for not attending play dates, birthday parties or family gatherings. His mother and father would try to encourage him to be more 'sociable' but they eventually gave up, thinking that Mohammed simply preferred his own company. His classmates described him as 'a bit of a loner', whereas his teachers used the word 'introvert' to describe his character.

Later in his school career, Mohammed found it difficult to summon up the courage to apply for a university place, especially as it meant that he would have to move out from his parents' home and into student accommodation. In his own mind, he had accepted that he was and would always be incapable of having a 'normal' social life. However, having dreamt of becoming an engineer since an early age, Mohammed was determined to continue his studies, which led him to apply for university. He ate all of his meals in his room because he could not bear the thought of other students staring at him in the dining hall. He often admired the confidence of his fellow students, who seemed to meet new people and develop friendships by the day. He felt ashamed and embarrassed about his inability to fit in at university and 'be normal'.

In the final year of his degree, one of Mohammed's tutors suggested that he might want to visit the student counsellor to talk about his fear of social situations. The tutor, who had a sister who experienced social anxiety, explained that talking to a professional might be helpful because the counsellor could give advice on how to beat his fears. Mohammed was initially reluctant to consider the tutor's suggestion as he did not really see how anyone could possibly help him change when the social awkwardness was deeply rooted in his personality. It also meant talking about his shyness, which he found embarrassing. The first time he visited the counsellor he felt sure that she would tell him that there was nothing she could do to help, which would have made him feel worse about himself. He recalls feeling slightly confused after his session, when his counsellor had told him that he was subject to a particular form of anxiety called a social anxiety disorder (SAD). She explained that this could be treated and that Mohammed could expect to learn a number of helpful skills that would eventually make him feel more confident during social situations. He felt a small sense of hope but also rather overwhelmed by what lay ahead and from talking about his difficulties; nonetheless, he committed himself to further sessions.

As we have seen, many people who experience social anxiety may feel that their fears of social situations are a part of who they are, and that they can't change the way they feel. This, along with feelings of shame, fear and embarrassment, can make a person reluctant to seek professional help. If this is the case, listen to your friend or relative's concerns if he or she is willing and motivated to share them, and encourage him or her to speak to a GP, who will be able to offer advice or encouragement to see a psychologist, counsellor or psychotherapist. You can also offer to speak to a professional on behalf of your friend to find out what will be the best way for him or her to seek further help. Of course, a book such as this one can provide insight and skills in dealing with the issue; do make sure that you do not put too much pressure on someone to seek help. It is important that people do this by their own choice and in their own time. Too much pressure can cause a person to feel even more anxious and therefore delay or even prevent treatment. Take a look at the following example:

Lucy, aged 43, had lost all of her confidence since giving up her work in the city to care for two children. She felt inadequate and boring when she was with other people, always thinking that she never really had anything to contribute. She gradually stopped accompanying her husband to business dinners and she rarely saw anyone who was not a close friend or family member. Her husband, Gary, really wanted to support Lucy, but at the same time found it frustrating having to attend business dinners on his own. He begged her to seek professional help, and sometimes he would ask her several times a week to consider this. He would often say that she should do it for their children. This made Lucy feel guilty and she became increasingly critical of her own skills as a mother, which in turn made her feel even more anxious. It was not until Lucy was able to point this out to Gary that he realized that his attempt to encourage her to seek help had caused her to feel even worse about herself.

If you take away just one thing from reading this chapter, please remember that encouraging someone who has social anxiety to seek professional help does not mean that either of you have failed. It may be that the most supportive thing we can do is to help our friends or relatives to recognize the huge step they have made in asking for help and to support them in telling their story to a GP, counsellor or psychologist.

The frustrating thing about social anxiety

When a close friend or partner has experienced social anxiety for a relatively long period of time, he or she may have developed several habits over the years that serve to reinforce it. Earlier chapters in this book show that unhelpful behaviours include avoiding social situations, withdrawing in social situations, talking only about certain topics because they feel safe, or using alcohol to quell one's nerves. These safety behaviours may actually increase or maintain anxiety. If this seems strange, you may find it helpful to read Chapter 4. During this time, it is possible that you have also developed certain ways of trying to help the person, some of which are less helpful and effective than others. A mother, for example, may ensure that her son is always accompanied by his older sibling when attending another child's birthday party because of his extreme shyness. She does this to protect her son from feeling anxious about going on his own to the party. Initially, this may have been a good way of encouraging the son to attend birthday parties. On the other hand, if he continues to be accompanied by an older sibling over a long period of time, he may never learn that he is capable of attending birthday parties and socializing on his own.

A similar situation could occur when a person offers to liaise with a colleague's boss because the colleague is afraid of making a mistake and being seen as stupid by her boss. The problem is that the colleague continues to really believe that she will make a fool of herself regardless of whether this is true or not. The belief is a fear and not necessarily a reflection of reality. She does not allow herself to be put in a situation where she can test out the idea that she may actually never make a fool of herself in front of her boss. Instead, she relies on another person to liaise with the boss because it immediately makes her feel less nervous. In the longer term, however, her social anxiety is perpetuated by avoidance enabled by her colleague.

A further example is when a husband spoke on behalf of his wife whenever they were at a social engagement. She became convinced that she could really embarrass herself by saying something uninteresting, which would make her feel more anxious. Although her husband was trying to help her feel more at ease by speaking on her behalf, he was also preventing her from building up her self-confidence, which she could achieve by exposure and engaging in social conversations.

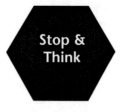

Stop & Think

Can you think of any habits you have developed that are helpful to your friend or relative? Are your actions helpful, or do they stop your friend from confronting his or her anxiety? If you discover that you have developed ways of supporting your friend that are not helpful, gradually stop this behaviour. This will ensure that you are not enabling him or her to use safety behaviours which are likely to reinforce the person's anxiety in the longer term. You may wish to speak to your friend first to explain what you are doing and why, so that the two of you can work out a plan on what is going to be the easiest way for you to stop reinforcing your friend's difficulties.

Learning to strike a balance between enabling avoidance and being sensitive to the need for progress is a difficult task for most people. It requires patience and understanding from both the person with social anxiety and those who are trying to give support. If you find yourself in a situation where a friend or relative is experiencing acute anxiety, stay calm and ask him or her to use the breathing exercises introduced in Chapter 6.

Seeing someone you care about in acute distress can be very upsetting and can leave you feeling helpless and scared yourself. Perhaps the first thing to remember is that acute anxiety generally doesn't last very long. Most people will calm down to a great extent within 30 minutes, although it may seem much longer to you. If you are responsible for someone in acute distress, reminding yourself that it will be over soon may help you stay calm. The most helpful thing you can do is keep the person safe, move him or her to somewhere more private and comfortable if you can, and offer to support your loved one in finding further sources of help if needed.

Supporting you as a helper

Another important thing to consider is that the effects of social anxiety can be as challenging to a partner, family member or friend as they are for the person who carries the burden of this fear. It is important to also consider support for yourself, as how you cope is likely to influence how the person with social anxiety copes, and vice versa. When it comes to coping with social anxiety, or indeed most other forms of psychological difficulty, the state of our family relationships as well as how our partners or close friends adapt to the situation may matter more to us than anything else. Where close relationships come to feel tense, strained, emotionally distant or volatile, these changes can tip the balance and make us susceptible to increased anxiety, depression and hopelessness, and even worse. An understanding of how relationships can be affected paves the way for more open communication and improved support, both of which have been linked to more favourable health outcomes.

As we have seen, helping someone deal with social anxiety cannot be prescriptive or formulaic, and depends on the needs of the person as well as the specific characteristics of his or her partner, friend or relative. There are a number of points to consider, however, such as learning as much as you can about the condition, not being afraid to ask someone what he or she needs, balancing the need to encourage with learning when you need to be patient and allow some avoidance to continue.

10

What to do if self-help isn't enough

Most of what we have covered in the book so far addresses self-help strategies, skills and techniques that you can apply to help you to understand and begin to overcome the fears you have come to associate with social situations. Hopefully, you will have already had some opportunity to try out some of these aids.

As we have already said right at the start of the book, there is no single 'one-size-fits-all' solution to the issue of social anxiety, and each individual will need to try a different range of approaches and solutions to be able to discover the one which works best for him or her. It is a form of trial-and-error experimentation, but since everything we have described is based on tried and tested and well-researched techniques, there should be at least some which are effective for you.

If you have gained some insight into the nature of social anxiety and shyness but do not yet feel confident in applying any of the techniques, do not despair! Social anxiety is one of many psychological difficulties that requires the right key to fit into the lock. It also requires time, persistence and patience in order to achieve satisfactory outcomes.

For some, the idea of obtaining the help and support that you may feel you need from friends, family members, work colleagues or professional helpers such as your GP, therapist, counsellor or psychologist can make you feel as if you are in a Catch-22 situation. Your social anxiety and feelings of embarrassment and/or shame may prevent you from speaking to other people in the first place! As we have seen elsewhere in the book, being able to share the issue with others can sometimes be an important step forward in overcoming it. Social anxiety is one of those difficulties that often makes seeking support from others very challenging: by speaking to others about your feelings you may be exposing yourself to further anxiety – just the very thing you were trying to avoid in the first place. That is why we have included this chapter, which addresses why progress may sometimes be slower than you had hoped or expected and what you can do about this. The contents of the chapter are also designed to reassure you that slower-than-expected progress is normal and does not necessarily indicate that you have a much more serious difficulty than you first thought.

Some reasons why progress may be slow

Below, you will find a list of the more common explanations of why you continue to experience difficulty with social anxiety. This is by no means an exhaustive or complete list, but it can serve as a checklist against which you can measure your own progress and ongoing difficulties. If you at least have some understanding of why you continue to struggle with your shyness, hopefully you can gain a deeper understanding of how it affects you and the ways modern psychological theory helps us in understanding how different people progress at different rates in their treatment.

This chapter will conclude with some suggestions as to what to do if the anxiety persists.

Working too hard at solutions that should work

Many readers will be familiar with the adage 'If you keep applying the same solution to the same problem, you will produce the same outcome.' This can be applied to most psychological difficulties, and social anxiety is no exception. If, for example, your attempted solution to social anxiety is avoidance, as we described earlier, this solution is unlikely to help you make appreciable progress with your difficulty. You are likely to experience some temporary relief or feel that you have coped with a difficult situation by avoiding it, but you will not have taken effective steps to overcome the underlying issue. As you worked through the previous chapters, you may have reduced the extent to which you avoid challenging situations. It is important to know, though, that avoidance can also extend to psychological interventions and techniques, as well as situations that make us anxious.

As we have described already in this book, there is a wide range of cognitive and behavioural techniques, skills and interventions that you can use in order to challenge and overcome social anxiety. However, if you avoid situations where you can test out the effectiveness of these or measure your progress, then they are merely textbook ideas. At some point, we need to move the ideas from the page or the laboratory into the real world and test how they work for us. This can sometimes be daunting, stressful or even emotionally too painful. If this is the case, we may need to go back a step or two so that we are not overwhelmed by our feelings.

With most psychological difficulties, it is preferable to take gradual, comfortable but determined steps forward and to gain confidence, rather than to take giant leaps and risk all. There is little point in escalating stress and anxiety to levels that feel unbearable. It may be necessary to try something else, or something less difficult. For example, if one attempted solution was to try to go to a party that you were fearing, but you had to leave the party early feeling significantly more stressed than before you set out, then perhaps you have attempted too big a first step. Once you have taken time to calm down and reflect, it may be worth scaling your next interventions back to starting a short conversation with the person sitting next to you in your local coffee shop. You may, for example, ask the time or whether the sweetener is on his or her table. Remind yourself that scaling back in this way does not mean you have 'failed'. You have had the courage to try and take a big step. That may have been too challenging and made you very anxious, but you will almost certainly have learnt something. But gaining confidence in small steps is arguably better than taking the giant leaps that would expose you to greater stress and anxiety and potentially put you off overcoming your difficulty.

In addition, if your thoughts about what you need to do leave you feeling emotionally vulnerable and upset, then it is perhaps time to go back to gaining a clearer understanding of these thoughts and to explore your fundamental fear about what it is you think could happen to you. It may be that your underlying fear of some catastrophic outcome (such as being laughed at, ridiculed or teased) is driving the anxiety. This may need further exploration and understanding and targeted interventions, and such feelings can sometimes be best dealt with by speaking to a qualified specialist such as a psychologist, counsellor or therapist.

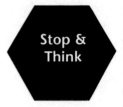

Stop & Think

Do you think that you may have been avoiding the psychological solutions most likely to help you? Can you explain why? Perhaps you have found some of the 'doing' techniques too challenging. Could that be because you have attempted to tackle something too difficult to start with and need to practise on smaller challenges first, or could it be that you need to take a little more time to work with the thoughts that drive your anxiety? Do you need someone to support you in your work, whether that's a friend or possibly a therapist?

Being able to work on these difficulties now

Motivational issues can also interfere with progress in psychological therapy generally. This is not to suggest that people who have psychological issues do not wish to overcome them – most of the time this is not the case. However, it is not always possible to give the time, focus and intensity needed in order to overcome the difficulty sufficiently. This may be because you are stressed or facing other difficulties in your life which can distract you from dealing with the matter in hand. Facing up to our psychological difficulties is rarely something we do independently from the presence of other issues in our lives. It may be that you are having a difficult time at work, for example, or are stressed by a child, or are facing health problems in the family.

Motivation may also be affected by the fact that we have lived with the anxiety for a long time. The effect of this is that we might have experienced reasonable coping with the difficulty in that we have found ways to avoid or manage – rather than solve – it. Sometimes being comfortable with our own solution to a difficulty, even though it is not a total solution, may interfere with efforts to overcome and cure the difficulty in the long run.

Motivational issues are also relevant in respect of the effort that is required. There is hardly any psychological issue any of us may encounter which does not require some effort if we are to overcome it. This is no different from gaining new skills in other areas of our lives. Do you remember the first time you learnt how to use a computer? Probably you were one of the many people who struggled to find the on/off button, accidentally deleted documents or got stuck transferring files from one folder to another. In psychological therapy, the initial stages can feel awkward, stressful and difficult to deal with. If you are struggling with making progress, it may be helpful to reflect on and consider your motivation to overcome the anxiety.

You might ask yourself a series of reflective questions to assess your circumstances and motivation, such as:

- Am I comfortable in my ways?
- Is it too much effort to make the necessary change?
- Do I have the energy, stamina or motivation to overcome this difficulty?
- Are the gains I could make outweighed by the comfort I feel staying as I am?
- Could anything else in my life be holding me back from making changes in my behaviour and dealing with uncomfortable and/ or stressful feelings?

If your answers to these questions show you that there may be obstacles in the way of working on the difficulties which caused you to read this book, it may be sensible to seek additional help by consulting a psychologist or therapist. Alternatively, it may be that, at least for now, the understanding you have gained by working through this book is enough.

Am I using the right 'new' solution for me?

Applying the wrong solution to the issue is similar to the first point that we have discussed. However, it may be that although this is a new solution you are applying, as opposed to an old one, it is still not the correct one that will help you achieve the necessary outcomes. If, for example, you keep challenging your negative automatic thoughts about social situations but fail to back this up with behavioural changes, your progress may be limited or temporary in extent. Conversely, if you change some of your behaviour without considering changes to some of your thoughts about experiencing social anxiety, your progress may be slow or limited. For example, if you avoid going to parties, you may try to reduce your anxiety by consuming copious amounts of alcohol in advance of the party. You may feel that alcohol might help you cope better with the stress of the situation. However, over-consumption of alcohol – as many readers will know – can inadvertently lead to disinhibited behaviour which, in turn, could draw the wrong sort of attention to yourself. It seems an easy solution, but it is potentially a self-defeating one. You may have more success if you work at challenging the anxious thoughts triggered by the situations you find difficult and then try to take small steps towards your ultimate goal.

What else is happening in your life now?

Psychological difficulties rarely exist in total isolation from other issues going on in our lives. We have partially addressed this point above; however, it is worth stressing that there may be what are termed 'cofactors' that interfere with your progress or maintain your social anxiety. If, for example, you are experiencing low mood or you have a physical health issue such as acne, a nervous twitch, blushing for a medical reason or another medical issue that affects your behaviour or appearance, such as Tourette's syndrome or an amputation, these difficulties may directly affect your social confidence and your feelings about being with other people or in a group of people.

Addressing social anxiety without first taking into account these additional issues or factors may hinder your progress. This is not to say that an individual who has acne needs to be completely free of any symptoms, or that a person with depression should be in perfect psychological shape before addressing social anxiety. It does mean, however, that such a person needs to take these additional factors into account when coming to understand his or her social anxiety.

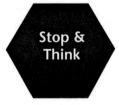

What's going on in your life right now? If you are facing some of the challenges we described above, it may be that you need to tackle these before working on your social anxiety. A qualified psychologist, therapist or counsellor can provide additional specialist help.

What is success?

Setting your sights on an instant and total cure to the difficulty of social anxiety may be a bridge too far. Experience tells us that the treatment of many fears and phobias can take time, and that progress may be gradual and incremental. If only there were a magic pill you could take and wake up the next day completely free of all symptoms! If you follow the standard psychological method using CBT, as described in this self-help book, you can expect progress to be gradual, sometimes a bit slow, but nonetheless incremental.

Treatment, whether with a psychologist, therapist or counsellor or through self-help, requires time, patience, perseverance and a measure of determination. There may be occasional setbacks, or at times it may feel as if you are playing a game of Snakes and Ladders: it can feel as if progress has been suddenly reversed, but then it quickly picks up steam again. Maintaining a positive outlook, a healthy dose of motivation and keeping the ideas described in this book in mind will help to keep you focused and on track.

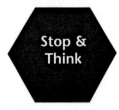

How will you know when you have successfully overcome your social anxiety? We cannot promise that you will never feel anxious in situations which challenge you. What would a realistic goal be? It might be to feel confident enough to join in some conversations at dinner parties or to be able to tell your manager about the problems you can see in his proposal. For example, when George started to work with his thoughts, as described in Chapter 8, he and his psychologist agreed that he would be successful if his anxiety reduced from 90/100 to 40/100.

When you set goals, it is important to make sure that they are appropriate for you and a realistic possibility. We often talk about SMART goals: targets which are Specific, Measurable, Achievable, Realistic and Time-limited. Here is a checklist which will help you make sure your goals are likely to help you successfully manage shyness:

- Be Specific – aim to be able to stay at a family party for two hours without your anxiety exceeding 60/100 rather than trying to cope with everything!
- Have a Measurable target – aim to reduce your anxiety at team meetings from 80/100 to 50/100 rather than just feeling better.
- Make sure it is Achievable and Realistic – to start with, aim to make a contribution to an interesting conversation next time you join friends, rather than aiming to present a lecture to 200 people.
- Put a Time limit on your efforts – plan when you will try things out, and if something doesn't help after two attempts rethink your approach.

Getting the right support

Involving others in your treatment and problem-solving can be enormously helpful. We do recognize, however, that someone who experiences social anxiety may find this especially difficult. It may be that the act of describing the issue to someone else is the first and most obvious stumbling block. It may be embarrassing or stressful to describe the anxiety to another person – who may not even be aware of it in the first place. Also, bringing yourself into close emotional proximity to others may just feel a step too far. Obviously we would encourage you to do this because, in our experience, trained and experienced specialists in this area will have already encountered many people who have similar difficulties. For them, this will not be new and nor will it be an uncomfortable situation. On the contrary, it is their job to help you with this difficulty and they should give you every encouragement along the way. Given that it is a treatable psychological condition, you can expect support and help in your efforts to overcome it.

Your starting point, if you decide to seek help from a trained specialist, could be that you have just read a book on overcoming social anxiety (this one!) and on the basis of what you have read you think you might be experiencing this difficulty. If you have been able to apply some of the ideas you have learnt in the book, you may also be able to describe why and how you feel the issue has come about and what you have done so far in order to overcome it. You could also possibly describe why you feel you are not making adequate progress in overcoming the difficulty. We recognize that taking the issue to someone else means facing up to it and verbalizing it to another person. Think of it as part of your therapy in that describing the difficulty and talking about it with another person is in itself therapeutic. Describing our difficulties is a major way in which we learn more about how they affect us and how we feel about them. It is an important next step in bringing about change.

A session with your GP, psychologist, counsellor or therapist will help to put you back on track by assessing the nature and extent of your anxiety and how best to treat it. This book can then act as a companion to that face-to-face treatment. You can use the book to help you think about homework exercises and in plotting your progress in overcoming social anxiety.

If you haven't made all the progress you would like

If you have decided that it is too difficult to act on some of the ideas suggested in this book at this time, or if you have made some progress but have not been able to take it far enough, you may become over-critical of yourself for not having 'cured' the anxiety. If you have worked through this book it is likely that you have already made some progress, so start by giving yourself credit for what you have achieved. Reading even parts of this book means that you have shown courage and motivation to take steps to overcome your social anxiety. Perhaps the act of buying the book was itself a recognition that there is an issue which you need to face. At the very least, you now have more information about the nature of social anxiety, which is a good start to overcoming it.

Remember the way in which we described how to challenge

negative thoughts about social anxiety earlier in this book (see Chapter 8)? Use those techniques to make more realistic challenges to any critical thoughts you may be having if you have found that you are not making the progress you would like. At the very least, you can congratulate yourself that you have started to face up to your anxiety.

Useful addresses

If you need more than can be offered by a self-help book, you may want to work with a psychologist or counsellor. We can be contacted via our website:
www.dccclinical.com.

Other sources of psychologists include the following:

British Association for Behavioural and Cognitive Psychotherapies (BABCP)
Imperial House
Hornby Street
Bury
Lancs BL9 5BN
Tel.: 0161 705 4304
Website: www.babcp.com

British Association for Counselling and Psychotherapy (BACP)
BACP House
15 St John's Business Park
Lutterworth
Leics LE17 4HB
Tel.: 01455 883300
Website: www.bacp.co.uk

The British Psychological Society (BPS)
St Andrew's House
48 Park Road East
Leicester LE1 7DR
Tel.: 0116 254 9568
Website: www.bps.org.uk

Health Professions Council
Park House
184 Kennington Park Road
London SE11 4BU
Tel.: 020 7582 0866
Website: www.hpc-uk.org

These associations all set standards for membership and their websites offer a search facility to find a therapist near you. If you want to know that a psychologist who has been recommended is registered with the

Health Professions Council in the UK, its website allows you to check this. Your GP will also be able to put you in touch with reputable local professionals.

Index